PRAISE FOR
ALZHEIMER'S MATTERS

Even as a neurologist who treats persons living with Alzheimer's and other dementias, I felt unprepared when thrust into the role of secondary caregiver for my father, Lester, after his diagnosis. Sure, I knew the epidemiology, pathophysiology, and clinical features of Alzheimer's. But I had little appreciation for the personal and emotional impact on caregivers who accompany their loved ones on this journey, and I felt ill-equipped to help my mother with the challenges of caregiving. In *Alzheimer's Matters*, Dr. Terri Baumgardner has provided precisely the kind of comprehensive resource my family needed at that time. What makes this book unique is its honesty and authenticity. Dr. Baumgardner gives encouragement and hope, yet does not shy away from describing the struggles she and her family faced in caring for her mother, Sally. When reading this book, one can sense someone walking alongside, helping to bear the burden, sharing the struggles, and rejoicing in the uplifts. There is something here for every caregiver. But healthcare providers who treat persons living with dementia also should read this book, and thereby grow their empathy and appreciation for the plight of caregivers.

—**Daniel C. Potts**, MD, FAAN
Neurologist, Tuscaloosa VA Medical Center
President, Cognitive Dynamics Foundation

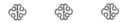

As a daughter, whose own mother lived with dementia for 30 years, I can say *Alzheimer's Matters* would have been helpful when my family started our journey. Dr. Baumgardner cuts a family's work way down as she has pulled together medical definitions, stages, testing, and more, along with options and supportive tools, combined with her personal experience. My guess is this book will become a resource book you will want to share within your inner circle.

—**Lori La Bey**, Founder & CEO of Alzheimer's Speaks

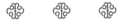

Alzheimer's Matters is an invaluable resource for caregivers of people with all forms of dementia. As an Industrial Gerontologist, I found this book to be an excellent comprehensive guide to helping caregivers during and through every stage of dementia. Terri includes the personal perspective of taking care of her mother, including the emotional and physical tolls on her mother and herself. Her book goes beyond the clinical presentation of the disease, providing a guide that gives readers a sense that they are not alone in this fight. On a personal level, I used this book as an insight into my own experiences with a relative in the early stages of vascular degeneration and dementia. *Alzheimer's Matters* takes the mystery out of caregiving and is an important book for all—especially as the population ages.

—**Lisa Park**, Ph.D., Industrial Gerontologist

This book provides valuable insight into the issues associated with an aging population that is experiencing memory decline associated with dementia. Terri's personal journey with her mother resonated with me as I began my journey with an aging parent. In addition to the emotional connection, it was comforting to have a guide to what is happening and where to turn for help. This is a unique book, as the author provides her own experiences and then takes the reader's hand in this uncertain world of diagnosis, treatment, and decline in an honest, but caring, way. When faced with the diagnosis of Alzheimer's or any dementia, reality quickly becomes surreal. Thanks to *Alzheimer's Matters*, there is a book and a community that can help chart the unknown.

—**Elaine C. Schwartz**, Esq.

Other than articles from the internet, this book is my first in-depth resource on Alzheimer's and dementia. Since I am the primary caregiver for my uncle who was recently diagnosed with dementia, this book has provided me excellent guidance into his care. The book is formulated in such a manner that it provides valuable information on other books, research, references, and trials, interspersed with a personal history. This helps one understand the disease so much better since one can relate to the various stages of the disease through the eyes of another caregiver.

The "What Next" section was very important to me at this stage of my uncle's care. It has helped me formulate our plan for his care. There is so much important information in this book that I have post-it notes guiding me back to sections that I feel are important and need to be revisited as I continue to care for my uncle.

—**Donna Chappel**, Business Owner & President

ALZHEIMER'S
MATTERS

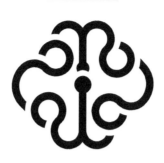

ALZHEIMER'S MATTERS

A Family Guide for Every Stage
of the Disease From Pre-diagnosis
to Death and Grieving

Terri L. Baumgardner, Ph.D.

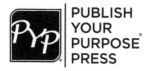

PUBLISH
YOUR
PURPOSE
PRESS

For permission requests, write to the publisher, addressed "Attention: Permissions Coordinator," at the address below.

Publish Your Purpose Press
141 Weston Street, #155
Hartford, CT, 06141

PUBLISH
YOUR
PURPOSE
PRESS

The opinions expressed by the Author are not necessarily those held by Publish Your Purpose Press.

Ordering Information: Quantity sales and special discounts are available on quantity purchases by corporations, associations, and others. For details, contact the publisher at orders@publishyour purposepress.com.

Edited by: Melissa Wuske and Karen Ang
Cover design by: Joan Cox
Typeset by: Medlar Publishing Solutions Pvt Ltd., India

Printed in the United States of America.
ISBN: 978-1-955985-18-5 (paperback)
ISBN: 978-1-955985-19-2 (hardcover)
ISBN: 978-1-955985-20-8 (ebook)

Library of Congress Control Number: 2021919041

First edition, November 2021.

Publish Your Purpose Press works with authors, and aspiring authors, who have a story to tell and a brand to build. Do you have a book idea you would like us to consider publishing? Please visit PublishYourPurposePress.com for more information.

This book is dedicated to my mother, Sally Ann Sarber Baumgardner, who taught me the most important life lessons. Through her example, I learned about love, kindness, lack of judgment, acceptance, forgiveness, sharing, happiness, humor, strength, humility, grace, sacrifice, enjoying every moment of life, and the importance of friends, family, and God. These are the lessons she learned from her mother, my grandmother Dorothy, who also suffered and died with Alzheimer's, but who—like my mom—was so much more than the disease. These are two women who lived well in this world. I am so grateful that they are my heritage, my family, my examples, my heart.

TABLE OF CONTENTS

PART ONE

"DO YOU MEAN ALZHEIMER'S?"
Understanding an Alzheimer's Diagnosis

PART TWO

"BE KIND AND BE STRONG."
Living with Alzheimer's Disease

PART THREE

"GIVE IT TO GOD."
The End of Life with Alzheimer's Disease

FOREWORD

As the founder of Alzheimer's Research and Treatment Center in Florida, I have been working with individuals with Alzheimer's disease and their loved ones for the past 26 years, serving as Principal Investigator on over 400 clinical trials for the treatment or prevention of this disease. As such, my staff and I see the impact of the disease firsthand on those who have it, and their loved ones. In addition—and similar to Dr. Baumgardner's family history—I also had a grandmother who suffered with Alzheimer's whom I cared for, and also lost several other family members to the disease.

Upon being referred to me by a mutual friend, I first met Terri when she visited the Alzheimer's Research and Treatment Center in Wellington, Florida. She was interested in talking about what we do there and sharing more about Alzheimer's Matters, the company she recently founded. She also wanted to get my feedback on her book. While I get requests similar to this on a fairly regular basis, I typically have to say no because of my time constraints in caring for my patients and their families. But, Dr. Baumgardner was persistent, and I knew from her background with a Ph.D. in Industrial/Organizational psychology and a master's in journalism, that she had likely approached the research and writing with scientific rigor and a keen eye. I was very pleased to see that I was right.

Once I started reading the book, I appreciated the way that she wrote it, with each chapter dealing with a phase of the disease, starting with her personal experience with her mother and then providing an overview of the research and resources available related to each stage. It was an honest telling and provided a strong depiction of what a family might expect to go through with this disease. Once I started reading about Terri's mother's story, I wanted to keep reading. I looked forward to the next chapter to see Terri's and her mom's next move (both good and bad), and her emotional feelings, which are clearly relayed in her writing.

Through this book, she conveys so much about what people might expect to go through at every stage of this disease. She opens up a window and allows the reader to look in on this very personal and emotional time. She emphasizes the importance of providing love, compassion, and empathy for those who have this awful disease, and working to bring them as much joy as possible each day. Unfortunately, there is still a great deal of negative stigma associated with Alzheimer's disease. Terri helps readers understand that there should not be, and—as with any disease—people who have Alzheimer's deserve dignity and every human right.

Beyond sharing the personal story, Terri makes sure that the reader is not left stranded, and provides information, research, resources, and guidance that can help in dealing with each stage of the disease. She has done her research to ensure that this book provides a solid and comprehensive overview of areas such as diagnosis, experimental trials, treatment, and care. She has talked with experts like myself, asked for our feedback, and made the book a better resource from it.

Anyone who has a loved one with Alzheimer's will benefit from reading this book—as will anyone who works in the field—because reading it will help them understand a family's experience and perspective.

David Watson, Psy.D.
Founder
Alzheimer's Research and Treatment Center

PREFACE

When my mother had cancer close to 15 years ago, my sister-in-law, brother, or I took her to every appointment. We were there with her for every chemotherapy treatment. We worked together as a family, with Mom at the center, battling against the non-Hodgkins lymphoma that invaded her body. Up until that point, it seemed like that was the fight of our lives.

Mom survived non-Hodgkins lymphoma and lived a decade free of that disease. She won that battle, but not the war.

On March 6, 2013, not even ten years after she was diagnosed with cancer, Mom was diagnosed with Alzheimer's disease.

This disease was different. It took Mom's mind so slowly at first, and then it took her body. Bit by bit, every human ability to function was gone until it stopped her breath.

Mom passed away on June 29, 2017, four years and four months after her diagnosis.

During most of that time, my husband and I lived with her, and I was her primary caregiver. I knew, as did my mother, that Alzheimer's disease was fatal. Years prior, we watched my mother's mother and two of her brothers die with the disease. It was my mother's worst fear. And I felt helpless.

All I knew to do was to love and to learn.

So, I strove to bring Mom as much joy as possible each day, and to never let her feel like a burden.

I also studied, read everything I could find on the topic, documented every doctor's visit, took notes, listened, and learned. When your loved one is going through Alzheimer's or another dementia, there is so much to learn at every stage of the disease that will inform so many actions and decisions. All of the information may be new to you. You may not know what your loved one might go through throughout the course of the disease, where to look for help, or how to decide on the best help. And, in many cases, you are solely responsible for making the decisions for your loved one, as this disease prevents them from participating in decisions when they are made.

This book is my effort to take what I learned—both about loving someone through this disease and about the knowledge that is important for people impacted by this disease—and share it.

Every chapter of the book represents a stage in dealing with the disease and begins with our very personal story. The personal experiences shared are not meant to imply that everyone will undergo the same, as I have been told by many medical professionals that no two instances of Alzheimer's disease are identical. But I believe that sharing the personal experiences throughout the book as honestly as possible is critically important, as fully honest depictions of the disease were lacking for me. In general, people who have not yet dealt with the disease do not seem to understand its true impact. Movies often romanticize the disease and leave people thinking that it has only to do with losing one's memory. Books often take a purely medical perspective, and do not address the personal and emotional journey.

The personal story that begins each chapter is mostly focused on the experience my mother and I had together with this illness. I have purposely not included a great deal of information about other family members, such as my brother, my sister, and their families. This is because I do not want to invade their privacy or speak for anyone else. I have shared everything that I am comfortable sharing and that I am fairly certain my mother would be comfortable with me sharing.

While every chapter begins with a personal story, it continues with a summary of the knowledge that is important for people who are dealing with this disease. The chapters end with a section titled "What Next?" with ideas for steps to take if you or your loved one is impacted by the disease. There is so much to know and so little time to learn it when you are caring for someone who has Alzheimer's. I hope this book will make this learning easier. While not meant to provide definitive or comprehensive medical information, it highlights information that I learned along the way from solid sources. At times, this book may suggest a bleak picture in terms of the support and options available for those impacted by the disease. To be sure, everyone will not have the same challenges as we did in areas such as finding the right caregiver, the right doctor, or the right experimental trial. I am conveying our specific challenges, but trying to do so honestly and being as vulnerable and open as I can in doing so.

This is a disease of losing one's mind, one's identity, and, eventually, every bodily function because as the brain goes, so does the body. Just think of that. What can possibly be more devastating?

My hope is that this book will help caregivers face this devastation with knowledge, compassion, confidence, and resilience.

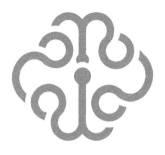

PART ONE

"DO YOU MEAN ALZHEIMER'S?"

Understanding an Alzheimer's Diagnosis

CHAPTER 1

PRE-DIAGNOSIS

When people say, "You have Alzheimer's," you have no idea what
Alzheimer's is ...
And you don't know what to expect.
—*Nancy Reagan*

Alzheimer's was my mother's greatest fear.

She saw her own mother regress and wither for years and then die from the disease in 1991 at the age of 76.

My mother's oldest brother was the next family victim of the disease. In 2006, at the age of 75, he died of Alzheimer's and pneumonia, which is a typical complication associated with Alzheimer's.

This loss was followed by several traumatic experiences for my mother, all within the span of a few years. She was involved in a car accident, concerned about her financial resources, and lost a new love who was very important to her. She had reunited with a man who she knew throughout her school years and, in her early seventies, found herself in love again. Near the time of Mom's diagnosis—for reasons known only to my mother and this man—he left to return to his home across the country.

Then, on June 4, 2012, my mother lost another brother—one who looked after her all of her life and who was also her best friend. He, too, died with Alzheimer's disease and with melanoma, which had spread throughout his body by the time he passed. During his illness, my mother traveled often between her home in Florida and his in Pennsylvania. She was there in his home at his passing.

The stress of watching her beloved brother suffer and die may have been too much for her to take. Less than a month after his death, Mom ended up in the emergency room with an incident of syncope, or fainting, with an unknown cause. A CT scan and an MRI of the brain were completed and both indicated "moderate atrophy," or degeneration of the brain, with no evidence of head trauma.

Looking back at the time prior to Mom's diagnosis of Alzheimer's disease, it is easier now to see the stress that was impacting her life. At the time, it seemed that each thing happened apart from the other events, and the connections between the events and their overarching impact were not as obvious as they are now. My mother also never complained of her problems. As many mothers do, she shielded her children from her own feelings of stress, grief, and pain—thus adding to the difficulty of seeing any changes that may have existed.

I am not sure now whether my mother ever really rebounded after her brother's death in 2012.

It turned out that she had reason to fear Alzheimer's.

By the time my uncle passed away with Alzheimer's in 2012, over 5.4 million Americans[1] and close to 35 million people worldwide were living with the disease.[2] Yet, even with a family history of the disease, I still knew so little about it. Today, I know much more.

In 2019, the number of Americans living with Alzheimer's has grown to 5.8 million,[3] and projections are that by 2050, this number could rise to 13.8 million.[4] Worldwide, in 2018, there were 50 million people living with

Alzheimer's or related dementia and, as the population ages, this number is projected to triple to 152 million by 2050.[5] Today, there are more people living with Alzheimer's worldwide than the population of Spain. In 2050, there will be more people living with the disease than the population of Russia!

So, what exactly is Alzheimer's?

The United States Department of Health and Human Services National Institute on Aging (NIA) defines Alzheimer's disease as an irreversible, ultimately fatal, progressive brain disorder that slowly destroys memory and thinking skills and, eventually, the ability to carry out the simplest tasks. In most people with the disease—those with the late-onset type—symptoms first appear in their mid-sixties. Early-onset Alzheimer's occurs between a person's thirties and mid-sixties and is very rare. Among older adults, Alzheimer's disease is the most common cause of dementia (a general term for loss of memory and other cognitive abilities serious enough to interfere with daily life).[6]

If you are a woman, African American, or Hispanic, it seems you are more, rather than less, likely to get Alzheimer's disease.[7] Almost two-thirds of Americans with Alzheimer's are women; older African Americans are about twice as likely to have Alzheimer's or other dementias as older whites; and some studies suggest that older Hispanics are about one and a half times as likely to have Alzheimer's or other dementias as older whites.

The personal impact of the disease spreads beyond the 50 million people who have Alzheimer's or related dementia. It also affects the families and friends of these people. In 2018, over 16 million family members and friends provided 18.5 billion hours of unpaid care to people with Alzheimer's and other dementias, at an economic value of $234 billion.[8]

The cost associated with unpaid care is just a portion of the financial impact. The total estimated worldwide cost of dementia in 2018 is $1 trillion. By 2030, the cost is projected to rise to $2 trillion.[9]

Republican Congressman Gus Bilirakis recently referred to Alzheimer's disease as one of the greatest threats to our nation's public health, harkening back to a characterization made by Dr. David Satcher, former surgeon general and director of the Centers for Disease Control and Prevention (CDC). Congressman Bilirakis added, "It is imperative that we work together to solve the problem ... Time is of the essence. The health of future generations and our nation's fiscal health is at stake."[10]

With what many consider to be inadequate funding for Alzheimer's and dementia over the last decades, it is not surprising that research progress has been slow. However, for decades now, researchers have known that two abnormal structures called plaques and tangles are characteristic of brains damaged by the disease. Plaques are deposits of a protein fragment called amyloid beta (or amyloid-β) that build up in the spaces between nerve cells. Tangles are twisted fibers of another protein called tau that build up inside cells.

The amyloid hypothesis, or the assumption that the accumulation of amyloid beta is the main cause of Alzheimer's disease, has dominated research in the field for more than 25 years. In recent years, though, the failures of several high-profile clinical trials of drugs targeting amyloid beta are a reason researchers are beginning to question the role of amyloid beta in the disease. In addition, more researchers are not settling with the conclusion that the plaques and tangles cause Alzheimer's. Instead, they are asking what causes the plaques and tangles to form in the first place, and then searching for solutions to prevent or reverse it. More recent research streams and experimental trials are examined more closely in Chapters 5 and 6.

While researchers are still investigating the root causes of Alzheimer's and dementia, the risk factors associated with the disease are better understood. The greatest known risk factor for Alzheimer's disease is increasing age. Of Americans ages 65 to 74, 3% have Alzheimer's. For those 75 to 84, 17% have Alzheimer's, and for those 85 and older, 32% have the disease. Of Americans who have Alzheimer's dementia, 81% are age 75 or older. One in three seniors dies with Alzheimer's or dementia.[11]

Having a family history of Alzheimer's is a second risk factor for the disease. Those who have a parent, brother, or sister with the disease are more likely to develop Alzheimer's. The risk increases if more than one family member has the illness. When diseases tend to run in families, heredity (genetics) or environmental factors—or both—may play a role.

Genetics represents a third major risk factor for the disease. Researchers have identified Alzheimer's genes in both of the two categories of genes— deterministic and risk genes—that influence whether a person develops a disease, as shown below.

Table 1.1.   Deterministic and Risk Genes

Definition	*Types*
Deterministic genes directly cause a disease, guaranteeing that anyone who inherits one will develop a disease.	Three, which are rare, accounting for less than 5% of Alzheimer's cases: • amyloid precursor protein (APP), on chromosome 21, discovered in 1987 • presenilin-1 (PS-1), on chromosome 14, identified in 1992 (variations in this gene are the most common cause of inherited Alzheimer's) • presenilin-2 (PS-2), on chromosome 1, discovered in 1993
Risk genes increase the likelihood of developing a disease but do not guarantee it will happen.	• Apolipoprotein E-e4 (APOE4) was the first risk gene identified, and it remains the gene with the strongest impact on risk. Everyone inherits a copy of some form of APOE from each parent. The APOE gene provides instructions for making a protein called apolipoprotein E. This protein combines with fats (lipids) in the body to form molecules called lipoproteins. Lipoproteins are responsible for packaging cholesterol and other fats and carrying them through the bloodstream. Maintaining normal levels of cholesterol is essential for the prevention of disorders that affect the heart and blood vessels (cardiovascular diseases), including heart attack and stroke. There are at least three slightly different versions (alleles) of the APOE gene. The major alleles are called e2, e3, and e4. The most common allele is e3, which is found in more than half of the general population. The e4 allele (APOE4) is the risk gene associated with Alzheimer's. If you inherit one copy of APOE4, your risk triples. If you have two copies, your risk is ten to fifteen times higher, though this is rare. But having APOE4 does not mean you will definitely develop Alzheimer's, nor does the absence of APOE4 mean that you will not develop Alzheimer's.

Genetic tests are available for both APOE4 and the rare genes that directly cause Alzheimer's. However, to date—outside of use in research studies—health professionals and Alzheimer's-related organizations have not generally recommended routine genetic testing for Alzheimer's disease. Concerns include that genetic testing can be difficult emotionally, provide inconclusive results, and cause practical difficulties.

While genetics, family history, and older age are the most recognized risk factors associated with Alzheimer's, more recently, researchers increasingly recognize that other factors, such as stress and lifestyle—including diet and exercise—play a role in the prevention or development of the disease. One study found that nine modifiable risk factors account for approximately 35% of all cases of dementia.[12] These nine modifiable risk factors are: early education up to age 15 years, hypertension, obesity, hearing loss in mid-life, depression, diabetes, physical inactivity, smoking, and low social contact in later life. While this is one study, there is an accumulation of research that suggests that some lifestyle interventions may contribute to dementia prevention, and that stress management may be the most important modifiable risk factor.[13] More information on modifiable risk factors and lifestyle interventions is included in Chapter 5.

What Next?

1. If you or your loved one has a family history associated with Alzheimer's, think carefully about the possibility of completing genetic testing. Many Alzheimer's-related organizations and health care providers do not currently recommend this, but it should be a very personal and well-thought-out decision. Consult with doctors and your loved ones, do more research, and seek genetic counseling, in order to make the right decision for you.

2. Most experts in the field of Alzheimer's today recognize that lifestyle interventions, including stress management, diet, and exercise are likely key contributors in preventing the disease. Obesity and diabetes

may be connected to inflammation of the brain, which is increasingly referenced as a factor in Alzheimer's. Working to maintain or improve good health, to reverse health issues such as obesity and diabetes, and to find positive ways to manage stress, will have benefits for the body but also for the brain.

CHAPTER 2

DIAGNOSTIC ASSESSMENT

The good physician treats the disease;
a great physician treats the patient who has the disease.
—*William Osler*

My mother was diagnosed with Alzheimer's disease on March 6, 2013. It was the worst day of my life—until the day that she died.

We had visited this neurologist's office once previously in January 2013 for some initial screening. As a follow-up to this first visit, the neurologist ordered an EEG and a neuropsychological evaluation. These were both completed in February 2013.

We returned to the office in March to get the results of the testing.

It was on this day that Mom and I sat in the lobby marred by faded, cheap, brass-framed photographs of landscapes and flowers and sunsets. I remember thinking on our first visit how dismal the lobby was. There was nothing redeemable about it.

We waited for more than an hour until we were told that the neurologist was delayed at the hospital for an emergency visit. We tried to talk of positive things.

I was afraid and I knew Mom was afraid. She did not say so, but that was Mom—protecting me from worrying or from feeling guilty that I had brought her here in the first place. I felt worried and guilty anyhow.

Finally, we were escorted back to the exam room. A young woman, not the neurologist, entered the room first and said that she was going to ask Mom some questions, explaining that they needed to ask these memory questions at every appointment.

"I'm determined to do much better this time," my mother said, referring to the earlier appointments in January and February, when the neurologist and neuropsychologist had asked her memory-related questions. Somehow, she had remembered the feeling of not doing well on the previous tests. Mom then told the woman how lovely she looked that day. Mom never missed an opportunity to compliment anyone.

The barrage of questions and instructions sounded something like this: "Sally, I'm going to say three words and ask you to remember them later. Bird. House. Tree. Now, what year is it? What is the date today? What are the names of your children? Now, look at this picture and draw it right next to it. Now, write your name on the line. Squeeze my hand. Now, stand up and walk to the wall and back. Now, what are the three words?"

Silence.

I was angry with this woman for putting my mother through this. Or was it me who was putting her through it?

Where was the neurologist? We were talking about a serious disease here, and we were worried about the results. We were worried about Alzheimer's.

As the young woman began reading from the report in her hands, she never said that dreaded word: Alzheimer's. She skipped quickly to the recommendations—come back in ten months, get cognitive therapy, take medication, drive only with someone else in the car, and get tested for driving again. Finally, the neurologist walked in.

Late and obviously harried, she glanced at each of our faces, tears on my mother's. She took the place of her colleague and began reading the results. I expected something more. We got something less.

She used the word "dementia."

"Do you mean Alzheimer's?" my mother asked so hesitantly that I knew she did not want to use that word either.

"Nothing is ever conclusive," the neurologist said. "You can't know with 100% certainty until ..."

She stopped herself. Then she returned to the recommendations. Why wasn't she trying to explain what they found and what it meant so that we understood? Why wasn't she sitting down next to my mom, looking my mom in the eyes, showing some kind of empathy? Instead, she continued standing the entire time, towering over my 5'2" mom, who was sitting crumpled on that hard-backed chair. She began emphasizing taking medication and having another driver's test. Mom did not want to hear that and started defended her driving skills.

"I'm a good driver, aren't I, Terri?"

I felt a physical ache in my heart. "Yes, you are a good driver, Mom. But you are starting to forget things. We need to know what to do."

My mother looked at me with love in her eyes. She was putting all of her faith and trust in me. I felt like I was not worthy of that. How was I going to do right by her in such an impossible situation?

As Mom and I walked to the car that day, holding hands (the way we always walked since the time it became clear that Mom was not comfortable on her own), I tried to say something positive, "Well, it's good that we did this so now we can know what we're dealing with."

"Yes, it's good," Mom responded—I knew it was more to protect me from feeling bad than because that was how she really felt.

As it was for my mother and me, the process of diagnosis can be extremely difficult for everyone involved. When you are going through it, you likely have an awareness that it is part of the early stages of that "long goodbye" that you have heard about. Your gut aches. Your mind searches for some detail to grasp—anything that might help. You need someone to hold your hand, to tell you it will all be okay, to protect you from what is coming. The trouble with this is that, in many cases, the person who always did this for you is the one who no longer can. It is now your turn to protect them.

Understanding the diagnosis process is one of the first steps to making sure a loved one gets the care and attention needed. In caring for your loved one, it is vital to understand how the diagnosis is reached.

Diagnostic Guidelines

Diagnostic criteria for Alzheimer's disease have been in place since 1984. At that time, diagnosis in living individuals was made as "possible" or "probable" based on clinical presentation and only classified as "definite" when specific histopathologic changes were found on autopsy.

Today, there is no one universally accepted protocol for diagnosing Alzheimer's disease. Three organizations have worked to develop, update, and publish their own sets of guidelines. The current version of each of these guidelines is outlined in Table 2.1.

The variations in the criteria for diagnosing Alzheimer's disease and the updating that occurs as more is learned about the disease can be confusing—even to medical professionals, let alone the average layperson. Nonetheless, the updating process is important. As such, the 2011 NIA-AA criteria were updated in 2018 for research purposes only (not as medical diagnostic guidelines).[1] The NIA-AA updates to the 2011 medical diagnostic criteria are currently in progress.

The 2018 NIA-AA research framework defines Alzheimer's disease not based on the symptoms or signs of the disease, but rather on the biomarkers found. The framework proposes three general groups of biomarkers (leaving room for other and future biomarkers): amyloid beta, tau, and neurodegeneration or neuronal injury. Only those with both the amyloid beta and tau biomarkers would be considered to have Alzheimer's disease.

Table 2.1.   Diagnostic Guidelines for Alzheimer's

National Institute of Aging—Alzheimer's Association (NIA-AA) 2011 guidelines	• Defines three stages of disease: ▪ *Preclinical*—brain changes may already be in progress, but significant clinical symptoms are not yet evident. ▪ *Mild cognitive impairment (MCI)*—symptoms of memory or other thinking problems are greater than normal for a person's age and education, but do not interfere with independence; people with MCI may or may not progress to the next stage. ▪ *Alzheimer's dementia*—symptoms of Alzheimer's are significant enough to impair independent functioning; the criteria for Alzheimer's dementia goes beyond memory loss as the first or only major symptom to recognize that other aspects of cognition, such as word-finding ability or judgment, may become impaired first. ▪ Recognizes the distinctions and associations between Alzheimer's and non-Alzheimer's dementias, as well as between Alzheimer's and disorders that may influence its development, such as vascular disease. • Recognizes the potential use of biomarkers—indicators of underlying brain disease—to diagnose Alzheimer's disease; however, the guidelines state that biomarkers are almost exclusively to be used in research rather than in a clinical medical setting involving patient care.
The International Working Group (IWG) for New Research Criteria for the Diagnosis of Alzheimer's Disease 2014 guidelines	• Requires the presence of cognitive symptoms plus biomarker evidence of physical pathology associated with Alzheimer's. This evidence could be either an abnormal amyloid PET study or an abnormal cerebral spinal fluid (CSF) testing (both will be described later in this chapter).
The American Psychiatric Association's *Diagnostic and Statistical Manual of Mental Disorders, Fifth Edition (DSM-5)* 2013 guidelines	• Distinct from above two guidelines, does not include reference to biomarkers. • Distinguishes between minor and major neurocognitive disorders with major showing a more dramatic decline in neurocognitive performance (shown through test performance or doctor evaluation) and cognitive deficits sufficient to interfere with independence.

The clinical or medical diagnostic framework, once finalized, should enable a more consistent evaluation process, which should benefit both practitioners and patients. Caregivers should understand the recommended guidelines and ask physicians about them, as needed.

More often than not, however, the patient and caregiver are unaware of the overarching criteria being used for evaluation. What they experience, though, are medical professionals using a combination of tools to diagnose the disease. Until there is a standardized clinical process for diagnosis, these methods and tools may vary from one professional to another. Currently, though, these tools typically include: obtaining a medical and family history from the individual and/or family members—including psychiatric history and history of cognitive and behavioral changes; conducting physical and neurologic examinations and cognitive and neuropsychological tests; and having the individual undergo blood tests, brain imaging, and other biomarker testing to rule out other potential causes of dementia symptoms, such as a tumor or certain vitamin deficiencies.

History Interviews

In the history interviews, one of the things that professionals look for is a family history of Alzheimer's. This history is an important factor of the diagnostic process.

In addition, in the history interviews, physicians look for indications of the initial warning signs of dementia. The Alzheimer's Association notes that because Alzheimer's changes typically begin in the part of the brain that affects learning, the most common early symptom of Alzheimer's is difficulty remembering newly learned information.

Alzheimer's Disease International (ADI), the international federation of Alzheimer associations around the world—including the Alzheimer's Association in the United States—summarizes the ten warning signs of dementia:

- Memory loss
- Difficulty performing familiar tasks
- Problems with language
- Disorientation to time and place
- Poor or decreased judgment

- Problems keeping track of things
- Misplacing things
- Changes in mood or behavior
- Trouble with images and spatial relationships
- Withdrawal from work and social activities

These changes tend to happen consistently over time, rather than intermittingly, and the person is unable to rectify the situation through methods like eventually recalling what they have forgotten.

It is often up to the people who spend the most time with the Alzheimer's afflicted person to notice these symptoms and report them to the doctor whenever it is time for a medical checkup. The person with Alzheimer's will not always recognize that there are any trends in their symptoms and may often not remember them in order to report accurately to the professional.

In addition, the person with Alzheimer's can demonstrate phenomenal skills in hiding their challenges from those around them, whether consciously or not. Perhaps the person does not remember the challenges and, therefore, denying them is natural.

Physical and Neurologic Exams

The medical workup is similar to a typical visit with a physician (e.g., review medications, listen to heart and lungs, collect blood or urine samples, etc.). During a neurological exam, the physician will closely evaluate the person for problems that may signal brain disorders other than Alzheimer's. The doctor will look for signs of small or large strokes, Parkinson's disease, brain tumors, fluid accumulation on the brain, and other illnesses that may impair memory or thinking. He or she will test reflexes, coordination, muscle tone and strength, eye movement, speech, and sensation. It is important to know that as a result of these exams, the physician may be able to identify reversible causes of any symptoms, which can then be proactively addressed and resolved. This is a major reason why anyone with concerns about their symptoms should complete these examinations as soon as possible.

Cognitive Tests

According to the Alzheimer's Association, two of the most commonly used mental/cognitive tests are the mini-mental state exam (MMSE) and the Mini-Cog© test.

The MMSE is an 11-question measure that tests five areas of cognitive function: orientation (to time and place), registration (of objects named), attention and calculation (spelling backward and counting by multiples), recall (of words), and language (following several commands). It takes only five to ten minutes to administer the test. The maximum MMSE score is 30 points. A score of 20 to 24 suggests mild dementia, 13 to 20 suggests moderate dementia, and less than 12 indicates severe dementia. On average, the MMSE score of a person with Alzheimer's declines about two to four points each year.

In the Mini-Cog© exam, a person is asked to remember and, a few minutes later, repeat the names of three common objects and draw a face of a clock showing all 12 numbers in the right places and a time specified by the examiner.

In a more extensive workup, the Wechsler Adult Intelligence Scale, Fourth Edition, (WAIS-IV) may also be used. It contains ten unique core subtests and five supplemental subtests that focus on four specific domains of intelligence: verbal comprehension, perceptual reasoning, working memory, and processing speed. The test also reports results for Full-Scale IQ (FSIQ) and General Ability Index (GAI).

Neuropsychological Tests

These tests help doctors determine if a person has dementia and if they're able to safely conduct daily tasks, such as driving and managing finances.

They provide as much information on what a person can still do as well as what may be lost. These tests can also evaluate if depression may be causing symptoms. The tests used may vary from doctor to doctor. The following table provides a summary of some of the common tests employed.

Table 2.2. Examples of tests used in diagnosing Alzheimer's

Assessment/Test	Use, Structure, Scoring, and Timing
Boston Naming Test (BNT)	Tests visual naming ability and consists of 60 line drawings of objects of graded difficulty, ranging from very common objects (e.g., a tree) to less familiar objects, such as an abacus; 35 to 45 minutes to administer
F-A-S	Assesses phonemic fluency (type of verbal fluency) by requesting an individual to orally produce as many words as possible that begin with the letters F, A, and S within a prescribed time frame, usually one minute
Animal Naming Test (ANT)	Aids in assessing general dementia; 60 seconds to name as many animals as possible
Test of Premorbid Functioning (TOPF)	Allows estimation of person's level of cognitive and memory functioning before the onset of injury or illness; 70 items; less than ten minutes to complete
Geriatric Depression Scale (GDS)	Facilitates assessment of depression in older adults; 30-item questionnaire in which participants are asked to respond by answering yes or no in reference to how they felt over the past week; a Short Form GDS consisting of 15 questions also exists; any positive score above 5 on the GDS Short Form should prompt an in-depth psychological assessment and evaluation for suicidality
Trail Making Test (Trails)	Measures attention, visual screening ability, processing speed, and overall cognitive functioning; it consists of two parts: TMT-A requires an individual to draw lines sequentially connecting 25 encircled numbers distributed on a sheet of paper; TMT-B is similar, except the person must alternate between numbers and letters (e.g., 1, A, 2, B, 3, C, etc.); the score on each part represents the amount of time required to complete the task

(continued)

Table 2.2.　Examples of tests used in diagnosing Alzheimer's *(continued)*

Assessment/Test	Use, Structure, Scoring, and Timing
Stroop Color and Word Test (Stroop)	Helps to differentiate between non-brain damaged and brain-damaged individuals; test-taker reads color words or names ink colors from different pages as quickly as possible within a time limit; the test yields three scores based on the number of items completed on each of the three stimulus sheets; five minutes to administer.
Repeatable Battery for the Assessment of Neuropsychological Status (RBANS)	Measures cognitive decline or improvement in immediate memory, visuospatial, constructional, language, attention, and delayed memory; 12 subtests; the RBANS index scores are converted to classifications including Very Superior, Superior, High Average, Average, Low Average, Borderline, and Extremely Low; 30 minutes

Brain Imaging, Lumbar Punctures, and Laboratory Testing

The brain imaging tests done for the diagnosis or exclusion of Alzheimer's disease include:

Computed Tomography (CT) Scan

A CT scan (or CAT scan) is a noninvasive diagnostic imaging procedure that uses special X-ray measurements to produce horizontal, or axial, images (often called slices) of the brain. CT scans often can reveal certain changes that are characteristic of Alzheimer's disease in its later stages. These changes include a reduction in the size of the brain (atrophy), widened indentations in the tissues, and enlargement of the fluid-filled chambers called cerebral ventricles.

Magnetic Resonance Imaging (MRI)

Magnetic resonance imaging (MRI) of the brain is a safe and painless test that uses a magnetic field and radio waves to produce detailed images of the brain and the brain stem. An MRI differs from a CT/CAT scan because it does not use radiation. MRI is beneficial in ruling out other causes of dementia, such as tumors or strokes. It also might help to show some physical changes in the brain that are associated with Alzheimer's disease.

Electroencephalography (EEG)

In an EEG, electrodes are placed on the scalp over several parts of the brain in order to detect and record patterns of electrical activity and check for abnormalities. This electrical activity can indicate cognitive dysfunction in part or all of the brain. Many patients with moderately severe to severe dementia of any sort have abnormal EEGs. An EEG may also be used to detect seizures, which occur in about 10% of Alzheimer's disease patients, as well as in many other disorders.

Positron Emission Tomography (PET) Scan

PET scanning is a three-dimensional imaging technique, utilizing the injection of a radioactive tracer that enables a doctor to examine the heart, brain, or other internal organs. PET scans can also show how the organs are functioning, unlike X-ray, CT, or MRI, which show only body structure. PET imaging can show the region of the brain that is causing a patient to have seizures and is useful in evaluating degenerative brain diseases, such as Alzheimer's, Huntington's, and Parkinson's. PET scans can show the difference in brain activity between a normal brain and one affected by Alzheimer's disease. They can also help differentiate Alzheimer's disease from other forms of dementia.

Amyloid Imaging

This is a special type of PET scan that shows deposits of amyloid, a protein, in the brain and provides a high degree of confidence in the diagnosis.

Before amyloid PET, these plaques could only be detected by examining the brain at autopsy. A positive test for amyloid does not mean someone has Alzheimer's, though its presence precedes the disease and increases the risk of progression. But a negative test definitively means a person does not have it. Individuals may opt to have this test done, but it is generally not covered by insurance and can cost several thousand dollars. In 2013, the Centers for Medicare & Medicaid Services (CMS) declined to cover the tests, citing insufficient evidence that they would make a difference for patients with a disease for which there is no cure and limited treatment available. Today, the most likely avenue for having this test completed is through participating in a clinical or experimental trial that includes the test as part of the examination.

Lumbar Puncture

In addition to these brain imaging tests, a lumbar puncture, also called a spinal tap, may be performed. This is an invasive procedure in which the fluid surrounding the spinal cord (called the cerebrospinal fluid or CSF) is withdrawn through a needle and examined in a laboratory. Testing the CSF can help the doctor diagnose disorders of the central nervous system that may involve the brain, spinal cord, or their coverings. CSF testing can identify protein related to Alzheimer's disease.

Other Laboratory Testing

Today, blood tests for predicting presence of brain amyloid pathology also exist. For example, companies like C2N Diagnostics have developed the APTUS™-Aβ42/40 test, which can predict if a patient is likely to have brain amyloidosis. Currently, this test is offered commercially for use in clinical trials and will soon be available as a test for clinical/medical use, according to the company's website.

Retinal imaging is also an important development for Alzheimer's detection. Companies such as RetiSpec have developed a patented technology that uses retinal imagery in synergy with machine-learning to allow for rapid, simple, and cost-effective identification of Alzheimer's biomarkers years before the emergence of clinical symptoms.

In addition, recent holistic approaches to diagnosing and treating Alzheimer's disease recommend comprehensive testing that goes beyond what has been used previously. In *The End of Alzheimer's: The First Program to Prevent and Reverse Cognitive Decline*, Dale E. Bredesen, MD, outlines all of the specific tests recommended in his ReCODE approach to determine a treatment protocol, including genetic testing, several blood tests, several tests of trophic support, toxin-related tests, metal testing, cognitive performance testing, brain imaging, sleep study, and microbiomes testing.[2] He refers to his comprehensive testing approach as a cognoscopy, which he recommends for anyone 45 years or older. He also clearly defines what results are indicative on every test. In terms of brain imaging, Bredesen recommends an MRI with volumetrics or, optionally, retinal imaging, both of which he describes in his book.

What Next?

1. See a specialist for a diagnosis as soon as possible when symptoms of Alzheimer's or other dementias are first noticed. There are real benefits to the person afflicted or to their loved ones in taking this step early. First, something other than Alzheimer's can be causing the symptoms and can sometimes be reversed and cured, depending on the cause. Second, even if Alzheimer's is the cause of symptoms, it can prompt a person to make critical lifestyle interventions, which may make a difference in disease progression. Third, many of the experimental trials require a person to be in early to mid-stages of the disease to participate. Being diagnosed sooner allows for participation in a trial that may help

with the symptoms and certainly benefit future generations. Fourth, early diagnosis can help prompt planning that a person needs to address before the symptoms become so progressed that the person cannot be involved in planning. Fifth, it is helpful to loved ones to understand what is happening so that they can be best positioned to assist.

2. Take extra care in selecting a specialist to see. This will often be a neurologist for diagnosis. Get as many recommendations as you can from people who have personal experience with the specialists. If you have any misgivings about the first specialist you meet with, try a second and a third, until you find one whom you trust. You and your loved one may be meeting with this specialist for years.

3. At some point, a single set of clinical practice guidelines for diagnosing Alzheimer's may be established. In the interim, the NIA-AA 2011 guidelines are expected to be updated. Watch for these updates. Be familiar with the guidelines and ask professionals what diagnostic criteria they are using.

4. If you are taking a loved one for diagnosis, help them understand as much as possible what they might expect with the diagnostic visit(s). It is very typical for people going for such a diagnosis to be very anxious about it. Anything you can do to lessen their stress and anxiety about the process is beneficial.

5. Understand that a medical visit for diagnosis may prompt the loss of driving privileges—if the person has not stopped driving already—and be prepared for this. States have various policies regarding physician reporting of drivers with dementia to the Department of Motor Vehicles (DMV) for testing. Some states have mandatory reporting policies, others have optional reporting policies, and some have no policy regarding this issue. In Florida, for example, "Any physician, person, or agency having knowledge of any licensed driver's or applicant's mental or physical disability to drive … is authorized to report such knowledge to the Department of Highway Safety and Motor Vehicles." Even if the person going for diagnosis is still capable of driving, this will change,

and having a doctor involved in a planned discussion at some point can be helpful.

6. Consider the possibility of biomarker testing (amyloid imaging) for the most definitive results regarding Alzheimer's disease. Talk with your specialist and loved ones about the option and its costs and benefits. The procedure is not currently covered by insurance, but is often included as part of participation in clinical or experimental trials.

CHAPTER 3

DIAGNOSTIC RESULTS

> Somehow, knowing that Alzheimer's is coming mocks all one's
> aspirations—to tell stories, to think through certain issues as only
> a novel can do, to be recognized for one's accomplishments and
> hard work—in a way that old familiar death does not.
> —*Jane Smiley*

Mom and I left the doctor's office on March 6, 2013 with a printout of her results. When we got home, I opened the report and started reading. Parts of it I read aloud to Mom, but she was not really listening. It seemed to me that she had forgotten that we were just at the doctor's office and the context of the visit. She seemed to have forgotten any mention of Alzheimer's.

I came to learn later, through my own study rather than through a conversation with a doctor, that certain Alzheimer's patients do not have a conscious awareness of their symptoms or that they have the disease—a condition called anosognosia. Mom was likely one of these patients. Along the way, I met others suffering from Alzheimer's who realized what was wrong and could talk about it in the beginning stages of the disease. Mom really did not and could not.

The Neuropsychological Evaluation Report was one component of the results, comprised of three sections. The first section included several subsections, which were primarily a recap of what we shared with the doctor, so there were very few surprises. The subsections were: Referral and Background, Medical History, Current Cognitive Complaints, Psychological History and Complaints, Social History, Academic/Vocational History, Behavioral Observations, and Tests Administered.

The second section of the report was titled Test Results. The tests that were part of Mom's evaluation were: Wechsler Adult Intelligence Scale (WAIS-IV), Boston Naming Test (BNT), F-A-S, Animal Naming Testing (ANT), Test of Premorbid Functioning (TOPF), Geriatric Depression Scale (GDS), Trail Making Test (Trails), Stroop Color and Word Test (Stroop), and Repeatable Battery for the Assessment of Neuropsychological Status (RBANS).

The neuropsychologist's report based on the testing was written around several areas of cognitive and emotional functioning, as shown in Table 3.1:

Table 3.1. Sections in a neuropsychologist's report of cognitive and emotional functioning

Estimated Premorbid Ability and Current Cognitive Functioning	*The TOPF results were used to provide an estimate of premorbid IQ. These were compared to current overall cognitive functioning, as reflected by RBANS Total Index Score.*
Intellectual Functioning	*This was based on WAIS-IV FSIQ and subscale results.*
Language Functioning	*Language functioning was based upon the BNT, FAS, and ANT results.*
Visuoconstructional Abilities	*This summary was based upon the Visuospatial/Constructional Index of the RBANS and Block Design subtest of the WAIS-IV.*
Executive Functioning	*Executive functioning was based upon Trails B and Stroop tests.*
Emotional Functioning	*This summary was based upon the GDS results.*

We came to find later that the MMSE would be administered again and again to Mom, as it provides a quick assessment of level of memory functioning. At the initial testing, Mom's MMSE score was 27 out of 30. A score of 24 or

lower is indicative of cognitive impairment. So, at that point, Mom was still doing fairly well with some aspects of memory. The MMSE results alone were not enough to diagnose Alzheimer's, but everything else in combination, including the family history, supported the diagnosis made by the neurologist.

The third section of the Neuropsychological Evaluation Report included a summary, conclusions, and recommendations. The conclusions section read, in part (SDAT in this summary refers to Senior Dementia of Alzheimer's Type):

> *Neuropsychological test results, together with history and clinical observation, are consistent with a diagnosis of dementia ...*
> *The patient's pattern of performance on testing, along with clinical observations of confusion and loss of instruction set during testing, and family history of Alzheimer's disease suggests a cortical process (i.e., SDAT).*

In addition to the Neuropsychological Evaluation Report, there was a separate summary report provided by the neurologist. A section of this report was titled "Plan."

The neurologist's plan was: driving evaluation, diet and exercise, prescription medication (Aricept, generic name donepezil, 5 milligrams for one month, then 10 milligrams), PET scan for additional imaging, and B12 supplement.

While neither the neuropsychologist nor the neurologist ever said the word "Alzheimer's," even when asked directly by Mom, the neurologist's summary report read: Diagnoses: Alzheimer's Disease (331.0), Syncope and Collapse (780.2) (the syncope notation referred to the fall Mom had in 2012).

It is important for anyone whose loved one is completing a diagnostic assessment to understand that the process is often anxiety-provoking to the person going through it. It can also feel demeaning, embarrassing, and unsettling.

Imagine a doctor asking you questions like, "What year is it?" or "What are your children's names?" or "What city are you in?" and you do not know the answers.

The questions keep coming. You still do not know the answers. You sit there wondering what is wrong with you. Why is this person trying to make you look stupid? Why are you just sitting there and letting it happen?

Knowing that these feelings may exist doesn't mean that anyone should avoid diagnosis, but should be used to ensure that everyone is as prepared as possible for what can, and often does, happen. It is important to understand that these feelings of embarrassment and anxiousness are among the many reasons that diagnosis often gets delayed. Those with a loved one going through the process need to have and show empathy.

In fact, as hard as it may be to believe, among individuals living with Alzheimer's disease and other dementias, evidence indicates that as many as 50% have not been diagnosed; and, of those diagnosed, only 33% are aware of the diagnosis.[1] The 2015 American Gerontological Society working group reported that "older adults are inadequately assessed for cognitive impairment during routine visits with their primary care providers."[2]

In high-income countries, only 20 to 50% of dementia cases are recognized and documented in primary care. In low- and middle-income countries, the treatment gap is greater, with one study in India suggesting 90% remain undiagnosed. "If these statistics are extrapolated to other countries worldwide, it suggests that approximately three quarters of people with dementia have not received a diagnosis and therefore do not have access to treatment, care, and organized support that getting a formal diagnosis can provide," notes Alzheimer's Disease International (ADI).[3]

Even among those who have received a formal diagnosis, it is important to understand that—while not the norm—misdiagnosis can occur. A 2016 study presented at the Alzheimer's Association International Conference (AAIC) revealed rates of misdiagnosis.[4] The researchers looked at inconsistencies between clinical and neuropathological diagnoses in 1,073 people from the National Alzheimer's Coordinating Center (NACC) database. (The NACC was established by the NIA in 1999 to facilitate collaborative research and to record the cumulative enrollment of the 29 NIA-funded Alzheimer's Disease Centers (ADCs) across the United States.)

The study revealed that in 78% of the cases studied, both a clinical diagnosis and autopsy confirmed the diagnosis of Alzheimer's using the NIA criteria. However, 11% were diagnosed with Alzheimer's in the clinic but on autopsy, did not have the brain changes necessary for an Alzheimer's diagnosis ("false positives," or falsely determined positive diagnosis for Alzheimer's). Some disease or condition other than Alzheimer's was causing their dementia. Another 11% had Alzheimer's changes in their brains on autopsy, but were not clinically diagnosed with Alzheimer's ("false negatives," or falsely determined conclusion that Alzheimer's is not present when, in fact, it is). The most common cause of a false positive clinical Alzheimer's diagnosis in this study was vascular pathology. The most common cause of a false negative diagnosis was dementia with Lewy bodies (discussed later in this chapter).

An additional 2017 scientific review in the *Neurology and Therapy Journal* reported a diagnostic accuracy of 77% for a clinical diagnosis of Alzheimer's disease, even among experts. The researchers concluded that the "historical medical evaluation of dementia due to Alzheimer's is inaccurate 25% of the time," "there is often a delay in diagnosis of 2 to 3 years," and that the diagnosis of AD has been, but should no longer, be, a diagnosis of exclusion."[5]

When dementia is present, there are both currently irreversible and potentially reversible causes. Potential reversible reasons for dementia include: depression, medication interaction, vitamin B-12 deficiency, infections, hormone or thyroid imbalances, malnutrition, and normal pressure hydrocephalus (NPH).

In addition to Alzheimer's, some of the most common irreversible reasons for dementia are shown in Table 3.2.

It is important to understand all possible alternative causes for dementia and for misdiagnosis of Alzheimer's disease so that advocates of the person

Table 3.2. Most common irreversible reasons for dementia

Vascular dementia	Vascular dementia results from conditions that damage your brain's blood vessels (e.g., strokes, diabetes, brain hemorrhage), reducing their ability to supply your brain with the amounts of nutrition and oxygen it needs to perform thought processes effectively. Most experts agree that it is the second most common cause of dementia after Alzheimer's disease, accounting for 5 to 10% of the cases.
Lewy body dementia (LBD)	LBD is a progressive dementia caused by abnormal microscopic deposits, called Lewy bodies, that damage the brain over time. Most experts agree it is the third most common type of progressive dementia after Alzheimer's and vascular dementia, accounting for 5 to 10% of cases. Lewy bodies are also found in Parkinson's disease and Alzheimer's disease.
Mixed dementia	This is when more than one type of dementia occurs simultaneously; the most common type is when Alzheimer's disease and vascular dementia coexist.
Frontotemporal dementia (FTD)	FTD is a group of disorders caused by progressive nerve cell loss in the brain's frontal lobes (the areas behind your forehead) or its temporal lobes (the regions behind your ears). Some people with frontotemporal dementia undergo dramatic changes in their personality and become socially inappropriate, impulsive, or emotionally indifferent, while others lose the ability to use language. FTD tends to occur at a younger age than does Alzheimer's disease, generally between the ages of 40 and 45.
Parkinson's disease	It is estimated that 50 to 80% of those with Parkinson's disease eventually develop dementia. The brain changes caused by Parkinson's disease (abnormal deposits of proteins called Lewy bodies) begin in a region that plays a key role in movement and later can spread to affect mental functions.
Creutzfeldt-Jakob disease (CJD)	CJD is the most common human form of a group of rare, fatal brain disorders known as prion diseases, in which misfolded prion protein destroys brain cells. CJD causes a type of dementia that gets worse unusually fast.
Huntington's disease (HD)	HD is a progressive brain disorder caused by a defective gene. This disease causes changes in the central area of the brain, which affect movement, mood, and thinking skills. Symptoms usually develop between ages 30 and 50.

(continued)

Table 3.2.   Most common irreversible reasons for dementia *(continued)*

Posterior cortical atrophy (PCA)	PCA refers to gradual and progressive degeneration of the outer layer of the brain (the cortex) in the part of the brain located in the back of the head (posterior). It is not known whether posterior cortical atrophy is a unique disease or a possible variant form of Alzheimer's disease. PCA onset is usually between the ages of 50 and 65.

experiencing dementia can ensure that all reasonable alternative causes are considered and ruled out. These advocates and care partners know the person better than any medical professional, and it is incumbent upon them to assertively represent the afflicted person, who likely is not able to adequately represent him or herself.

Identifying the stage of the disease progression is another aspect of the diagnostic process. Table 3.3 provides a summary of the three stages of Alzheimer's identified by the National Institute on Aging.[6]

Table 3.3.   Three stages of Alzheimer's

Stage	Individuals Experience Difficulties and Symptoms Including:
Mild Alzheimer's Disease (Early Stage)	• Memory loss • Poor judgment leading to bad decisions • Loss of spontaneity and sense of initiative • Taking longer to complete normal daily tasks • Repeating questions • Trouble handling money and paying bills • Wandering and getting lost • Losing things or misplacing them in odd places • Mood and personality changes • Increased anxiety and/or aggression
Moderate Alzheimer's Disease (Middle Stage)	• Increased memory loss and confusion • Inability to learn new things • Difficulty with language and problems with reading, writing, and working with numbers • Difficulty organizing thoughts and thinking logically • Shortened attention span • Problems coping with new situations

(continued)

33

Table 3.3. Three stages of Alzheimer's *(continued)*

Stage	Individuals Experience Difficulties and Symptoms Including:
	• Difficulty carrying out multistep tasks, such as getting dressed • Problems recognizing friends and family • Hallucinations, delusions, and paranoia • Impulsive behavior such as undressing at inappropriate times or places or using vulgar language • Inappropriate outbursts of anger • Restlessness, agitation, anxiety, tearfulness, wandering—especially in the late afternoon or evening • Repetitive statements or movements, occasional muscle twitches
Severe Alzheimer's Disease (Late Stage)	• Inability to communicate • Weight loss • Seizures • Skin infections • Difficulty swallowing • Groaning, moaning, or grunting • Increased sleep • Loss of bowel and bladder control

*Adapted from National Institute on Aging website at www.nia.nih.gov.

A more detailed staging method was developed by Dr. Barry Reisberg (variations are referred to as the Global Deterioration Scale or GDS, and the Functional Assessment Staging Test or FAST). This staging method is used by professionals and caregivers around the world to identify what stage of the disease a person is in. Stages 1 through 3 are the pre-dementia stages. Stages 4 through 7 are the dementia stages. Stage 5 represents the point at which an individual can no longer survive without assistance. This stage is recognized as the "moderate dementia" stage in other models. Developers of this staging method note that Alzheimer's disease always progresses through the scale in order, although there are other dementia conditions that do not and with which patients might skip stages.

Alzheimer's patients and their caregivers may often first learn of the FAST and GDS stages when they are beginning to consider hospice care, but it can be helpful to know of these earlier. The scales have been used for many years to describe Medicare beneficiaries with Alzheimer's disease and a prognosis of six months or less. Normally, patients in hospice care for Alzheimer's are in Stage 7, experiencing profound levels of difficulty communicating and moving independently.

The FAST stages are summarized below.

Stage	Stage Name	Characteristic
1	Normal Aging	No deficits whatsoever
2	Possible Mild Cognitive Impairment	Subjective functional deficit
3	Mild Cognitive Impairment	Objective functional deficit interferes with a person's most complex tasks
4	Mild Dementia	Instrumental Activities of Daily Living (IADLs) become affected, such as bill paying, cooking, cleaning, traveling
5	Moderate Dementia	Needs help selecting proper attire
6a	Moderately Severe Dementia	Needs help putting on clothes
6b	Moderately Severe Dementia	Needs help bathing
6c	Moderately Severe Dementia	Needs help toileting
6d	Moderately Severe Dementia	Urinary incontinence
6e	Moderately Severe Dementia	Fecal incontinence
7a	Severe Dementia	Speaks 5–6 words during day
7b	Severe Dementia	Speaks only one word clearly
7c	Severe Dementia	Can no longer walk
7d	Severe Dementia	Can no longer sit up
7e	Severe Dementia	Can no longer smile
7f	Severe Dementia	Can no longer hold up head

The full version of the scale also provides expected untreated duration of each stage, mental age of person afflicted in each state, and expected MMSE score during each stage. Those with Alzheimer's and their caregivers should inquire with their medical specialist about these staging models and get professional assistance in understanding the models. Also, visit the Fisher Center for Alzheimer's Research Foundation website (https://www.alzinfo. org/understand-alzheimers/clinical-stages-of-alzheimers/) to learn more.[7]

What Next?

1. Ask for and maintain copies of all medical records and documentation. While you may never need to refer to them, it is just a smart practice.
2. Ask as many questions as needed to understand exactly what each test is showing and how conclusions are reached.
3. Be familiar with both the reversible and irreversible causes of dementia, and work with the specialist(s) to ensure that causes other than Alzheimer's have been ruled out.
4. Reference the FAST scale as needed. While often used related to determining if it is time for hospice care, it is a good reference tool to help understand the progression of the disease process.
5. After diagnosis, talk with the person diagnosed if possible, other family members, and professionals as needed, to determine what needs to be communicated and to whom. There should be no embarrassment or stigma associated with communicating information about this disease. However, even the person diagnosed may not want anyone else to know about their disease. Try to talk with him or her as openly as possible. Establish a plan with those who need to be involved.
6. When you do talk with friends and family members about the diagnosis, it is likely that they will ask how they can help. Be prepared to answer the question and to be as specific as possible. For example, you might tell someone, "It will mean a lot if you can come and visit every week, just for an hour or so. A routine for the same day and time every week would be helpful if that will work."

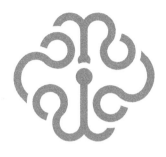

PART TWO

"BE KIND AND BE STRONG."

Living with Alzheimer's Disease

CHAPTER 4

MY BEST FRIEND, EMPATHY, AND LOVE

In my mother's house there was happiness,
I wrapped myself in it—was my chrysalis—
As my life unfolds, see a pattern through,
of you protecting me and I protecting you.
—*Corrine Bailey Rae, the song, "Butterfly"*

Initially, when writing this book, I did not intend to include this chapter that shares a little more about Mom—apart from the experience with her illness. That changed when I read the recent edition of the book The Best Friend's Approach to Dementia Care *by Virginia Bell and David Troxel. It reminded me of how important to the care process it is to know who my mom was. So, it seemed like a natural extension for readers to know something more about who Mom was in her life—long before Alzheimer's disease—in order to better understand the impact of the disease. The following note from Mom, shown in Figure 4.1, is a good example of her expressions of love for her children and grandchildren.*

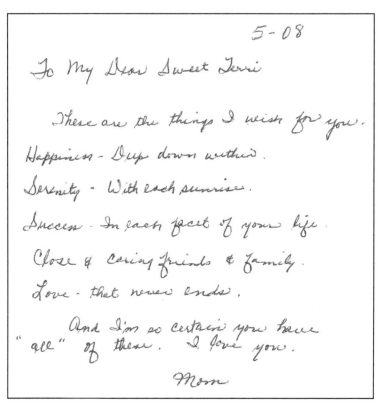

5-08

To My Dear Sweet Terri

These are the things I wish for you.
Happiness - Deep down within.
Serenity - With each sunrise.
Success - In each facet of your life.
Close & caring friends & family.
Love - that never ends.

And I'm so certain you have
" all " of these. I love you.
                    Mom

Figure 4.1.   A note from Mom in a journal she gave me years before her illness.

One day, shortly after Mom's diagnosis, I asked her, "What is your philosophy for life, Mom?"

I don't know why I asked it. In part, I was trying to ask as many questions as I could in order to soak up all of Mom's wisdom before it was no longer possible. Mom was not one to simultaneously offer up words of wisdom and sage advice anyhow. Even when you might try to pull it out of her, she resisted. She did not want to impose her point of view on anyone. Nor would she ever judge anyone. No matter the person's indiscretion, she would not give voice to a bad thought—if she had one.

On this day, she surprised me by how quickly she answered, as her communication skills were already declining a bit, her confusion was growing, and the question was not an easy one.

"Be kind and be strong," she said with no hesitation in the gentle voice I was so accustomed to hearing.

"Really? I never knew that before, Mom."

That was the first time I had ever heard Mom say that, but when she did, it made my heart ache. There was nothing that she could have said that would have described more perfectly how she lived her life. I could see through the fog that day to how that simple phrase had guided everything she ever did or ever said.

Mom fell in love with my dad when she was in ninth grade. They married soon after Mom graduated, and she stood steadfastly by his side for more than 30 years. She stayed at home taking care of her children for the first 11 or so years. One of the worst times of Mom's life was likely her divorce. Since she grew up in an age when most things revolved around husband and family, I did not know how Mom was going to make it through this trauma. But she did—with strength and dignity. While the early years were filled with tears and fears, soon she had a group of friends around her and they did everything together. Mom was happy.

When her first grandchild, my brother's daughter, Randi Elyse, was born, she was even happier. By the time her second grandchild, Jamie Alexis, was born, there was no keeping her away. She sold her home in Pennsylvania and moved to Florida where my brother had just moved with his young family. Mom moved into their small home with them where she slept in Jamie's room with her— forming the foundation for what would become one of life's great loves.

When Mom moved into her own home, she still spent every moment she could with her grandchildren and also opened her home to every visitor. We all joked that she ran a bed-and-breakfast. When you checked in, you did not want to leave—there was such a feeling of warmth and love in my mother's home.

Mom was always smiling. She said hello to everyone and made friends so easily. She said the funniest things, often so unexpectedly. She followed the stocks; played mahjong and canasta with friends; bought a teal blue BMW convertible and drove it on A1A with the top down and her baseball cap on, while singing along to Norah Jones or Corinne Bailey Rae; and she traveled whenever and wherever she could. She loved music more than anyone I've known.

Even during Mom's illness, she stood by her philosophy of being kind and being strong. While there were many hard times for her, she still extended her love and gratitude to others. She started conversations until she no longer could. She was gracious, caring, and genuinely loving, and she showed those around her how to be all of these things.

She was brave and strong. She survived a divorce. She fought a battle with cancer and won. She stood up against her worst fear, Alzheimer's, with grace. I remember so clearly one of the times when a home health aide was giving Mom a bed bath. It was late in Mom's illness, and sometimes even small movements hurt. Mom was not talking very much at all at this point, but at the end of the bath, she said, "Thank you." The aide, who knew Mom well, looked at Mom with tears in her eyes and said, "Only you, Sally." There were so many instances at the end of her illness when I knew Mom was in unbearable pain, and she closed her eyes and bravely bore it.

People who have cared for a loved one with Alzheimer's have likely found that some stigma still exists. They may have watched people talk to their loved one and, when the response does not make sense, the person turns to them with a look that suggests, "What in the world?" or even worse. Then they stop talking and turn away.

Even friends and family can disappear from the life of the person with Alzheimer's. They often rationalize why by saying things like, "She does not know who I am anymore, so it doesn't matter if I visit or not. It's too difficult to be with him. I don't know what to say or do. I can't just come over and sit there; I'm not someone who can just sit."

What people should understand is that those afflicted with Alzheimer's and other dementias still feel love and respond to it. It can be in the form of just sitting with the person or holding his or her hand or telling stories, even when the person cannot engage in the conversation. When people with

Alzheimer's are still able to have conversations, they may verbalize that they do not understand why their friends and family do not visit more. Whether others realize it or not, they are needed.

Alzheimer's may, in fact, be the loneliest disease. The person with Alzheimer's loses his or her connection to friends—not only in their minds, but often physically, as well. Often, the person and the primary caregiver spend an extraordinary amount of time alone with each other, because the support system that was there in the good times is often gone in the bad times. Even family members cannot deal with some of the challenges of the disease and become less present.

It can be very difficult to care for someone with Alzheimer's, but it is important to remember that they are the same someone who you have always loved and the same person who may have even spent a lifetime caring for you. People can say things like, "She's not the same person anymore. The person she was is gone." But "she" is the same person she always was, regardless of how the disease has impacted her. It's vital that caregivers make the conscious choice to care for her as such.

A few authors have written about the importance of love and care for those afflicted with Alzheimer's and dementia. These may be some of the most important books about the disease ever written.

The Best Friends Approach to Dementia Care is a standard for many who have experienced Alzheimer's or other dementias in their lives. The authors, Bell and Troxel, trademarked the Best Friends™ philosophy and approach to care and the widely used Dementia Bill of Rights, shown in Figure 4.2.[1]

The Best Friends approach to dementia care requires understanding a person, and its precepts should be followed by anyone dealing with Alzheimer's and dementia. It also requires demonstrating respect and, essentially, giving love. The authors refer to a caregiver's personality, affection, patience, and heart as their "knack," and they note that it is this knack that counts more than anything else in dementia care. What they refer to as the knack is really just about giving love and the understanding, patience, and empathy that come with that.

DEMENTIA BILL of RIGHTS

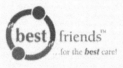

Every person diagnosed with Alzheimer's disease or other dementia deserves:

- To be informed of one's diagnosis
- To have appropriate, ongoing medical care
- To be treated as an adult, listened to, and afforded respect for one's feelings and point of view
- To be with individuals who know one's life story, including cultural and spiritual traditions
- To experience meaningful engagement throughout the day
- To live in a safe and stimulating environment
- To be outdoors on a regular basis
- To be free from psychotropic medications whenever possible
- To have welcomed physical contact, including hugging, caressing, and handholding
- To be an advocate for oneself and for others
- To be part of a local, global, or online community
- To have care partners well trained in dementia care

The Best Friends™ Dementia Bill of Rights by Virginia Bell & David Troxel. Copyright © 2013 Health Professions Press, Inc.

Figure 4.2.   Reprinted by permission.

The importance of love in the life of someone afflicted with Alzheimer's rings clearly through the words of Deborah Barr, Edward G. Shaw, and Gary Chapman in their book, *Keeping Love Alive as Memories Fade: The 5 Love Languages and the Alzheimer's Journey.* They say:

> Our most basic emotional need is not to fall in love but to
> be genuinely loved by another, to know a love that grows
> out of reason and choice, not instinct. I need to be loved by

someone who chooses to love me, who sees in me something worth loving. That kind of love requires effort and discipline. It is the choice to expend energy in an effort to benefit the other person, knowing that if his or her life is enriched by your effort, you too will find a sense of satisfaction—the satisfaction of having genuinely loved another ... [When] love is the attitude that says, "... I choose to look out for your interests" ... the one who chooses to love will find appropriate ways to express that decision.[2]

The authors continue to say that a word for this kind of love does not exist in English, but does exist in Hebrew. The word in Hebrew, they say, is *hesed* (HEH-sed). Author Lois Tverberg described the meaning of the word as follows: "*hesed* acts out of unswerving loyalty ... *hesed* is a love that can be counted on ... It's not about the thrill of romance, but the security of faithfulness ... *hesed* is not just a feeling but an action. It intervenes on behalf of loved ones and comes to their rescue."[3]

Person-Centered Care

The ideas of these authors are not the first references to the importance of love and person- and relational-centered approaches to interacting with people with Alzheimer's and other dementias. Person-centered care concepts originate as far back as 1949 in the foundational work of Carl Rogers and his approach to client-centered psychology.[4]

In 1997, Tom Kitwood wrote a book titled, *Dementia Reconsidered: The Person Comes First.*[5] In it, he discussed how individuals living with dementia have an enduring sense of self and they maintain feelings, preferences, and personality characteristics until the end of life. Kitwood's writing in this book is substantive, going beyond even what many of today's proponents of person-centered care discuss, and was far ahead of its time. Kitwood even talks about the struggles he had leading up to writing his book, noting that he wanted to use the phrase the "social psychology of dementia" and develop it in detail. He notes that social and interpersonal factors either add to the difficulties arising from neurological impairment or help to lessen their effects. In very many cases, he says, "we find that the process of dementia is also the story of a tragic inadequacy of our culture ... our medical system and our general way of life."[6] He continues, "If personhood appears to have been undermined, is any of that a consequence of the ineptitude of others, who have all their cognitive powers intact? If uniqueness has faded into a grey oblivion, how far is it because those around have not developed the empathy that is necessary, or their ability to relate in a truly personal way?"[7]

Today, a variation on Kitwood's person- and relational-centered care practices is accepted as the gold standard for health care by the World Health Organization (WHO)[8] and the Institute of Medicine.[9] The Organization for Economic Cooperation and Development said providing person-centered, coordinated care is one of the most pressing challenges facing health systems today, but it is "even more crucial for people with dementia, who have complex needs but limited ability to navigate complex health and social care systems."[10] The organization continued to say that dementia is one of the most misunderstood conditions in the developed world.

Over 20 years after Kitwood applied person-centered care concepts specifically to dementia care, "Alzheimer's Association Dementia Care Practice Recommendations" were published, with person-centered care as the foundation.[11] The Dementia Care Practice Recommendations illustrate the goals of quality dementia care in the following areas: person-centered care; detection and diagnosis; assessment and care planning; medical management; information, education, and support; ongoing care for behavioral and psychological symptoms of dementia and support for activities of daily living; staffing; supportive and therapeutic environments; and transitions and coordination of services.

The following practice recommendations are at the core of person-centered care:[12]

1. Know the unique and complete person, including his or her values, beliefs, interests, abilities, likes, and dislikes—both past and present.
2. Recognize and accept the person's reality; see the world from his or her perspective.
3. Identify and support ongoing opportunities for meaningful engagement.
4. Build and nurture authentic, caring, and respectful relationships that concentrate on the interaction, not the task.
5. Create and maintain a supportive community for individuals, families, and staff.
6. Evaluate care practices regularly, using tools available to assess person-centered care practices, and make appropriate changes.

The Alzheimer's Association provides specific suggestions related to every facet of their dementia care practice recommendations, which can be found on their website.[13] In seeking or receiving long-term care services for someone afflicted with Alzheimer's, know these recommendations and inquire with organizations and professionals about how they implement them. In the early stages, being familiar with the recommendations may help people with Alzheimer's understand and communicate their needs.

"The quality of dementia care rendered to individuals and families is contingent upon the quality of assessment and care planning, and the degree to which those processes are person-centered," say Sheila Molony, Ann Kolanowski, Kimberly Van Haitsma, and Kate Rooney, the authors of the article titled, "Person-Centered Assessment and Care Planning."[14] They go on to note that regular, comprehensive assessment is recommended at the time of initial diagnosis and interim reassessments are recommended in all settings at least every six months. The first priority is to detect issues that detract from quality of life or prevent the person with dementia from living fully. This includes detection of hidden medical illness or pain or sources of excess disability and assessment of the degree of engagement in enjoyable activities. The presence of caregiver challenges should also be assessed. More frequent reassessment is indicated in the context of recent medication changes, changes in health or behavior, living alone, driving, unstable or multiple conditions, bothersome symptoms, care partner stress, individual or care partner health concerns, recent hospitalization, or emergency department visits. The care partner's well-being and ability to provide support commensurate with the person's needs may also change over time. A person-centered approach will tailor the frequency of assessment to the individual and family situation.

Every person living with Alzheimer's and dementia needs the kind of person-centered care described above. When a person gives this kind of love and care, he or she expects nothing in return, but in fact, in the midst of this terrible disease, he or she can be rewarded. In giving, they receive.

While it feels almost blasphemous to say it … perhaps even such a horrendous disease such as Alzheimer's has something huge to offer—if only people can learn how to love through it.

What Next?

1. Read everything you can on person- and relational-centered care and inform those involved in the care process about it.
2. Make an effort to invite people to come and visit with the person struggling with Alzheimer's. They might be very unsure about how to handle this, so offer advice in advance for what they can do or say to help make the visit a nice one. For example, they can ask the person if they would like to go for a walk and take a short walk with them. Or they can ask them if they would like to listen to music and then play some music for them. Or go to a park together. Or lay by a pool. Many of the things that the person with Alzheimer's used to enjoy are likely things that he or she still enjoys if they have the capability, even though it might take gentle prompting.
3. If you are caring for a loved one with Alzheimer's, make an effort to take them to places where they can be with other people who know them and love them, or even to see new people. As long as you are with your

loved one, any anxiety from being with new people should be lessened for them.

4. Help identify and implement activities that your loved one may find engaging. As a primary caregiver, you know more about what these things might be than anyone else. In addition, the things that the person with Alzheimer's enjoys may be very different now than before having the disease. For example, just because they were very social before the disease does not mean that they will be comfortable in social settings after the disease. You can try things out if you think it isn't harmful for the person in any way. In addition, you might modify activities to make them easier for the person to enjoy. For example, you might arrange social activities but be with your loved one for these activities to make them more comfortable. It is a matter of finding out what might work best for you and your loved one.

5. As a person who loves someone with Alzheimer's, do what you can to educate others about the disease. There is still so much that people do not understand.

CHAPTER 5

TREATMENT

I often hear people say that a person suffering from Alzheimer's is not the person they knew. I wonder to myself, *Who are they then?*
—*Bob DeMarco, founder of Alzheimer's Reading Room*

I always thought that treatment and care were one in the same when it came to an illness or disease. That was not the case with respect to Mom's Alzheimer's disease.

This is the way that her treatment proceeded: a visit with the neurologist, some quick assessment of how far her disease had progressed from the last appointment, assessment of how the medication was working and if changing it seemed necessary, and scheduling the next appointment, usually for six months later. The treatment focus was on medication. There was nothing that I might consider a long-term holistic approach to care for a person with a fatal illness, at least for us, and at least until the point when we met Mom's hospice team (discussed in Chapter 8).

When we visited the original neurologist in March 2013 for Mom's diagnostic results, the treatment plan included a driving evaluation, diet and exercise, starting to take Aricept (generic name, donepezil), a PET scan, and B12 supplement. After the visit, Mom started receiving B12 supplement shots from her primary care doctor and started on Aricept. After a few weeks, she stopped taking Aricept because she was having stomach problems from it.

At the six-month point, in September 2013, we went to a new neurologist so that he could review the original results, provide a second opinion, and give his recommendations. This neurologist started by saying that Mom's memory problems could be due to three things. The biggest concern he noted was the hereditary nature of the disease and the history in the family. He also noted that it was possible that depression played some role, due to the traumatic events that occurred in 2012, the year prior to Mom's diagnosis—including the death of her beloved brother. Finally, he said that three of the medications Mom was taking (prescribed by her diabetes doctor) were shown to affect memory: gabapentin, simvastatin, and metformin.

He added that, as far as conducting further testing for diagnosis, there were four simple tests used for diagnosing memory problems and Alzheimer's. He noted that Mom had all of these and that the blood work, EEG and MRI all looked fine. Further, the results from the neuropsychology exam were known to be 90% accurate and the results for Mom were consistent with Alzheimer's disease. He said that the only other test that could be done was an amyloid PET scan—costing around $3,000 or more and not covered by insurance. He did not recommend this step, as he thought we had other steps to take first. Mom's next appointment was scheduled for November. In the interim, she would stop taking the gabapentin, monitoring for any effects from stopping, and try the Aricept again.

A few weeks after this visit, Mom stopped taking Aricept again as she was still having stomach problems. This time, the doctor prescribed the Exelon patch for her (another drug for treating dementia, its generic name is rivastigmine), which she used for some time. She eventually stopped using that when it seemed like the disease had progressed past the point of it helping at all, though it was difficult to know because Mom could never tell you, and you also had no idea how *progressed the disease would have been without the drug. When Mom stopped using the Exelon patch, the neurologist prescribed memantine (Namenda), which Mom took until the last months of her life.*

Almost a year after Mom's initial diagnosis, in February 2014, we had our third visit with this neurologist. During the period of time from November 2013 to near the end of Mom's life, we saw the neurologist about every six months for a quick assessment, check on medication, and any updates.

Despite the fact that this neurologist did not recommend it, Mom had the amyloid PET scan on March 13, 2014. We received a disk copy of the imaging and a report of the results, which was a few paragraphs long, with the last part saying: "Impression—The study is positive for cortical uptake consistent with the clinical diagnosis of Alzheimer's disease."

The disk results were provided with no explanation. The disk contained several files and file folders. One file folder contained 841 images in gray scale and in color; one image is shown in Figure 5.1. Mom's neurologist never reviewed the scans with us, only the conclusion. Later, when Mom tried participating in a clinical trial, we shared the file with the neurologist there. He sorted through the images but spent very little time looking at them. When asked to explain what he saw in one of the images, he quickly commented on the red versus yellow colors, but then said he needed to return to the exam room where Mom was waiting. I never understood why there was so little time and explanation devoted to the amyloid PET results. It was confusing and odd to me that we spent thousands of dollars to have the test completed, and all that was offered afterward was a one-page summary with one sentence confirming the Alzheimer's diagnosis. I speculated that maybe because the test was so new, and likely few people complete it because of the costs, that even specialists were not very comfortable with reading, interpreting, or explaining the results. I imagined that those trained with the technology were the ones who knew best how to interpret the results. However, when I asked the laboratory that completed the test if someone there could walk me through some of the results, I was told that the laboratory did not do that— that it was up to Mom's neurologist to do that with us.

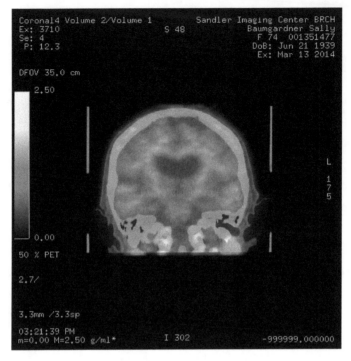

Figure 5.1. One of the images from Mom's amyloid PET scan.

When I first came upon Dr. Bredesen's 2017 book *The End of Alzheimer's: The First Program to Prevent and Reverse Cognitive Decline*, the title alone left me feeling optimistic for those with Alzheimer's disease and their loved ones.[1] I came to understand that his book and others with similar titles presented more holistic approaches to the disease than the diagnosis and drug treatment approaches I knew about. Dr. Bredesen's book provided a comprehensive medical explanation of the causes of Alzheimer's disease, according to his research, and a very extensive protocol that he noted had been shown to work in his practice to prevent and even reverse cognitive decline.

Dr. Bredesen, trained as a medical doctor at Duke University Medical Center and the founding president and CEO of the Buck Institute for

Research on Aging, was, however, despite the title of the book, personally cautious about conveying that his approach would definitively end this awful disease. In an interview with the website, "being patient," on September 4, 2019, he said that the title was not his idea, but his publisher's, and that he wanted to call it "Wit's End," reflective of researchers being at their wits' end trying to figure out what's going on with Alzheimer's, as well as what's happening to your brain when you have Alzheimer's.[2] Readers should take the same cautious approach in considering Bredesen's research. But, those impacted by the disease should consider it and make their own judgments. At the core of Bredesen's research is the big question: Is amyloid beta the cause of the disease, or simply a by-product or result?

Dr. Bredesen's book begins with discussing the current state of treatment of the disease as a sad one. But it was one I knew was very reflective of my mother's experience. He discusses how people often do not seek medical care because they have been told there is nothing that can be done. They fear things like the loss of their driver's license, the stigma of a diagnosis, and the inability to obtain long-term care insurance if diagnosed with a fatal disease. In addition, he notes that many primary care providers often do not refer patients to memory clinics, since they have been taught that there is no truly effective therapy. Therefore, they typically simply start patients on donepezil (Aricept), often without a firm diagnosis. Finally, specialists often put the patients through hours of stressful neuropsychological testing, expensive imaging, and repeated spinal taps and then have little or nothing to offer therapeutically.

In the 2017 book written by Dean Sherzai, MD, and Ayesha Sherzai, MD titled, *The Alzheimer's Solution: A Breakthrough Program to Prevent and Reverse the Symptoms of Cognitive Decline at Every Age*, the authors note that almost all of the Alzheimer's research is disease-based, meaning that scientists focus on developing a cure in the form of a single drug versus a more holistic therapeutic approach. Despite this focus, of the 244 compounds that were tested in a total of 413 clinical trials, between 2002 and 2012, only one new drug was approved: memantine (Namenda).[3]

To date, the U.S. Food and Drug Administration (FDA) has approved six medications for the treatment of Alzheimer's symptoms, shown in Table 5.1. The first drug currently used to treat Alzheimer's was approved in 1996; the last entirely new drug (rather than a combination of existing drugs), Aducanumab (brand name Aduhelm™), was approved very recently,

Table 5.1.   FDA approved medications for Alzheimer's

Generic Name	Brand Name	Approved For AD Stage	Additional Information
Aducanumab	Aduhelm™	Approved for Alzheimer's; results to date mainly for mild stage	Approval in 2021, so future results will follow
Donepezil	Aricept®	All stages; primarily used for mild to moderate	These drugs are referred to as cholinesterase inhibitors. They block the action of an enzyme called acetylcholinesterase, which breaks down acetylcholine (a brain chemical believed to be important for memory and thinking) to an inactive form.
Galantamine	Razadyne®	Mild to moderate	
Rivastigmine	Exelon®	Mild to moderate	
Memantine	Namenda®	Moderate to severe	This drug is referred to as an NMDA receptor antagonist. It works by changing the amount of a brain chemical called glutamate, which plays a role in learning and memory. Brain cells in people with Alzheimer's disease give off too much glutamate. Namenda keeps the levels of that chemical in check.
Memantine + Donepezil	Namzaric®	Moderate to severe	Works through a combination of both methods described above.

in 2021. None of these drugs cure the disease. Aducanumab, an intravenous (IV) infusion therapy that actually targets removing beta-amyloid from the brain, is the first treatment that research suggests may delay clinical decline. The other drugs treat the cognitive symptoms of Alzheimer's, such as memory and thinking.

Possible side effects of Aducanumab are ARIA (e.g., swelling in the brain), headache and fall; of Memantine are headache, constipation, confusion and dizziness; of Donepezil, Galantamine, and Rivastigmine are nausea, vomiting, loss of appetite, muscle cramps, and increased frequency of bowel movements. Namzaric®, since it combines the two drugs of Memantine and Donepezil, has the possible side effects of both.

Beyond the drugs already in use for Alzheimer's treatment, as of 2018, there were 112 agents (drugs) in the Alzheimer's disease drug development pipeline, according to an annual review of the clinicaltrials.gov database.4 Clinicaltrials.gov is a comprehensive U.S. government database of all clinical or experimental drug trials conducted in the United States. The database allows for anyone to track or locate human clinical trial research by disease and by phase of the research.

The phases involved in all human clinical trials include:

- Phase I, which usually includes a small number of healthy volunteers (20 to 100) for the purpose of determining the effects of the drug (or in some cases, device) on humans, including side effects;
- Phase II involves several hundred patients, can last up to two years, and consists of one randomized group of patients receiving the experimental drug and the second randomized "control" group receiving a standard treatment or placebo (generally, these trials are "blinded" with neither the patient nor researcher knowing who is in each group);
- Phase III involves randomized and blinded testing in several hundred to several thousand patients, often over several years, after which FDA approval for marketing a drug is possible; and

- Phase IV is conducted after approval for consumer sales and results of this phase of trials can lead to a drug being taken off the market or restrictions of use being placed on the drug.

In 2018, across all clinical trials related to Alzheimer's, 57% were sponsored by the biopharma industry. Thirty-two percent were sponsored by academic medical centers (with funding from National Institutes of Health, industry, or other entities) and the remainder by others.[5]

In contrast to the prevailing direction of drug research, Dr. Bredesen's book discusses the importance of new approaches related to Alzheimer's and dementia research. Bredesen bemoaned the state of the industry, noting that in 2011, he proposed the first comprehensive trial for Alzheimer's disease but that the institutional review boards (IRBs) denied permission for the trial, noting that clinical trials are designed to test a single variable such as a drug, but not multiple components simultaneously. "The standard avenues by which scientific discoveries become medical therapies had failed us—and had failed Alzheimer's patients," said Bredesen.[6]

Bredesen's recent book contains a thorough explanation, based on his research and study, of what he sees happening in the brain that results in an overabundance of plaques and tangles in the first place. Bredesen says that "Alzheimer's arises when the brain responds as it should to certain threats … [it] is what happens when the brain tries to protect itself from three metabolic and toxic threats: inflammation (from infection, diet, or other causes); decline and shortage of supportive nutrients, hormones, and other brain-supporting molecules; and toxic substances such as metals or biotoxins (poisons produced by microbes such as molds)."[7]

Simplified, Bredesen's research notes that there are subtypes of Alzheimer's, depending upon which of the threats a person's brain is experiencing: Type 1 is inflammatory (hot); Type 2 is atrophic (cold); Type 3 is toxic (vile). The protocol for treatment, prevention, reversal, and even cure, he says, is specific to each subtype; which subtype a person has is identifiable through testing. He calls the protocol ReCODE (for reversal of cognitive decline, outlined at length in his book). Bredesen advocates strongly for thorough testing, including APOE4 genetic testing, to even begin to understand what is happening in each person's brain (e.g., inflammation, lack of nutrients) and then to personalize the ReCODE approach needed.

Bredesen breaks from the typical Alzheimer's research in several ways. First, he argues that Alzheimer's is not a singular disease, but rather three syndromes depending upon whether the brain is experiencing Type 1-, Type 2-, or Type 3-related threats. There are different contributors or causes to each of these types, with 36 contributors in total. Second, no single drug will address the combination of contributors to the disease, therefore, the existing single-pill approach to treatment cannot be expected to succeed. Third, he posits that the three threats to the brain that result in Type 1, 2, or 3 are the causes of Alzheimer's and its associated plaques and tangles. This is in contrast to decades of research focused on the plaques and tangles as the cause of the disease. "Since the 1980s most neurobiologists have treated this basic idea, called the amyloid hypothesis, as dogma," he says. "Just as tragic as the blinkered adherence to the amyloid hypothesis is mainstream medicine's assumption that Alzheimer's is a single disease."[8]

Another author, Richard Furman, MD, a vascular surgeon, builds a case for the link between Alzheimer's and vascular dementia, sharing research findings supporting that it is now generally agreed that the two rarely occur in isolation but rather coexist. This is what is called mixed dementia. In his 2018 book, *Defeating Dementia: What You Can Do to Prevent Alzheimer's and Other Forms of Dementia*,[9] Furman notes that disease of the arteries in three areas of the body can have an effect on the brain: the arteries of the heart; the arteries that feed the brain, especially the carotid arteries in the neck (disease or plaque in these arteries is called atherosclerosis); and the small arteries in the brain (disease of these arteries is called cerebrovascular disease).

Furman concludes that finding a cure for Alzheimer's won't happen, because once brain cells die, they cannot be brought back to life. Since the process is irreversible, prevention is crucial and the health of the arteries is a key player that can be controlled in the fight against Alzheimer's through controlling these five factors: high cholesterol, sedentary lifestyle, excess weight, high blood pressure, and diabetes. This, of course, is best accomplished through a healthy diet, maintaining the ideal weight, and exercising. Furman's Prescription for Life diet emphasizes fruits and vegetables, whole-grain cereals, peas, beans, nuts, pasta, fish, and olive or canola oil. The foods to avoid are red meat, cheese, cream, butter, and fried foods—each high in saturated fat.

The 2017 book by Dean Sherzai, MD, and Ayesha Sherzai, MD, *The Alzheimer's Solution*, also supports the critical role of a healthy lifestyle in preventing Alzheimer's. The authors summarize that there are four interconnected processes responsible for the degeneration in Alzheimer's: inflammation—chronic inflammation of the brain caused by irritants, such as high-sugar diets or unmitigated stress; oxidation—the brain has special cells and molecules for breaking down and neutralizing free radicals (resulting from oxidation) that are damaged over time from things like poor diet and lack of exercise; glucose dysregulation—the system responsible for maintaining glucose often begins to falter with age and poor diets, having significant consequences; and lipid dysregulation—the improper clearance and processing of cholesterol and other lipids leads to vascular disease (a risk factor for dementia) and the formation of amyloid plaques.[10]

A comparative reading of both the Sherzais' book and Bredesen's book reveals a great deal of overlap in the identification of causes of Alzheimer's, beyond just referring to the build-up of amyloid plaques and tau tangles in the brain. The Sherzai research has resulted in a protocol for treatment and reversal of Alzheimer's called the NEURO (nutrition, exercise, unwind, restore, and optimize) plan. Like Bredesen's ReCODE protocol, it is a very holistic approach. It places the greatest emphasis on nutrition.

In his book, Bredesen references the birth of functional medicine, in which a physician determines the root causes of illnesses and treats all contributing factors. Functional Medicine, as defined by the Institute of Functional Medicine (IFM), is a systems biology-based approach that focuses on identifying and addressing the root cause of disease. Each symptom or differential diagnosis may be one of many contributing to an individual's illness, and a diagnosis can be the result of more than one cause. For example, depression can be caused by many different factors, including inflammation. Likewise, a cause such as inflammation may lead to a number of different diagnoses, including depression. The precise manifestation of each cause depends on the individual's genes, environment, and lifestyle, and only treatments that address the right cause will have lasting benefit beyond symptom suppression.

Even a quick review of the literature on functional medicine reveals that the field has its skeptics. David Gorski, MD, PhD, managing editor of *Science-Based Medicine*, wrote an article in 2016 titled, "Functional medicine: The ultimate misnomer in the world of integrative medicine." In it, he said, "The problem with 'functional medicine' is that at its core it is close to being as nonsensical as the more 'obvious' forms of quackery. It just hides it better, given the number of fancy-sounding laboratory tests."[11]

For years, even the American Academy of Family Physicians (AAFP) shared at least some skepticism about functional medicine, placing a moratorium on awarding any AAFP credit to activities and sessions on the topic. Then, in September 2017, the AAFP Credit System issued a call for comment on functional medicine to AAFP members. The request for feedback included a call for evidence on functional medicine's efficacy in the application of family medicine and any additional supporting evidence and/or literature. The information received was objectively reviewed and summarized in a report by a third party. That information, along with several literature reviews and results from the AAFP Member Survey, informed the decision to lift the moratorium on awarding any AAFP continuing education credits related to functional medicine education.

For now, the drug therapy treatment options do not cure, prevent, or reverse the progression of Alzheimer's disease. The most they might do is to slow the progression of the disease. The functional medicine approach to Alzheimer's disease seems like a more holistic approach that still has more than its share of skeptics.

However, what traditional medical professionals and functional medical practitioners seem to agree on is that lifestyle factors, such as diet, exercise, and stress management are much more important than originally thought. In the "Alzheimer's Disease International (ADI) World Alzheimer's Report 2018—The State of the Art of Dementia Research: New Frontiers," renowned researchers put forward this perspective.[12] Miia Kivipelto, a professor in clinical geriatrics at the Karolinska Institute in Stockholm, Sweden, and a senior geriatrician at the Karolinska University Hospital, was one of the first people in the world to identify the link between lifestyle and dementia. She led the FINGER study, the world's first large multidimensional study of lifestyle interventions, and believes that at least a third of Alzheimer's disease is related to factors that can be influenced.

According to the ADI report, Kivipelto is now helping to run international versions of FINGER adapted to different cultures, diets, and settings. The one in the United States, which will be run with Maria Carrillo, chief science officer at the Alzheimer's Association, is called POINTER. There are also versions in China, Singapore, and Australia. Kivipelto, who is also currently working with the World Health Organization (WHO) on risk reduction guidelines, says that it is too early to say whether the program affects amyloid beta levels in the brain, but she is hopeful.

It is in the hands of each person impacted by Alzheimer's and those who care for them to be as informed as possible about potential treatment options, and then decide how to move forward. It will feel hopeless at times, to be sure. But the field seems to be changing dramatically even as this book is being written, and real hope could be closer than many realize.

What Next?

1. Search for neurologists and other specialists (e.g., neuropsychologists) who can and do keep you informed about available treatment drugs, interactions, experimental drugs and trial options, and novel treatment ideas and options. Ask questions about options you have read about

that the specialist may not bring up. Bring information to the specialist, as you can, and ask for his or her opinion.

2. Read any new books and publications that come out on preventing, treating, or even curing Alzheimer's disease. Some of the approaches written about in new publications are not talked about on the typical websites you might go to for information. This could be because they are often considered novel and without sufficient typical clinical evidence to support them. If you feel strongly about an approach, though, keep digging into it. No medical professional cares more about your loved one than you, so remember that you are your loved one's best advocate. Push for what you believe and, at the same time, be open to contradictory research and scientific evidence to the contrary.

3. Much of what you read currently about Alzheimer's prevention will discuss the importance of lifestyle, diet, and stress management. Many recommend following a Mediterranean-style diet and a regular exercise regimen. Improving diet and exercise will help in overall health, including brain health, and can eliminate factors such as high cholesterol, diabetes, or inflammation, which may be linked to the onset of Alzheimer's.

4. Some of the newer research advocates a complete as possible understanding of your current health measures to determine your baseline and your risks, and then implementing a plan to proactively address any risks. Ignoring or delaying the option of having more complete health data for yourself will not change that data. It is better to understand your baseline and risk data, so that you can begin working to impact it for the good.

CHAPTER 6

EXPERIMENTAL TRIALS

Hopelessness has surprised me with patience.
—*Margaret J. Wheatley*

At one point, when meeting with Mom's regular neurologist, he mentioned a local doctor who was conducting experimental trials. We visited this doctor afterward to see if Mom could participate in any of these trials.

When we first met this doctor, he said with exasperation, "Why didn't any of the doctors you've seen recommend this sooner?" He explained that Mom could be too far along in her disease process for participation in most of the trials he was conducting.

We came to find out that each trial has criteria that a patient must meet to be able to participate. There were only one or two trials being conducted there at the time that Mom could even qualify for because her disease was too progressed.

During Mom's initial visit to this doctor in August 2015, she completed some testing with the purpose of further determining her eligibility for any of the trials. She took the Mini Mental State Exam (MMSE) again. This time, her score was 11 out of 30. When she took it two years earlier when she was diagnosed, her score was 27 out of 30. Among other errors, she could not name the year correctly (she answered 1967) or the season (she answered September), or the county or city we were in (she did not answer). She could not repeat, "No ifs, ands, or buts," or write a sentence or copy the design on the page.

In December 2015, Mom completed additional screening related to a particular experimental trial. Among several other tests, Mom completed the MMSE-2 and scored 11 out of 30 again—again unable to name the year, repeat three words after a pause, or copy a design on the page. When asked to repeat the three words after a pause, Mom said, "Can you repeat that to me? I can't remember."

In early 2016, Mom began participation in a Phase II study for the drug bryostatin 1 (the protocol number for the study was NTRP101-202). The study sought to enroll 150 moderately severe to severe Alzheimer's disease subjects, who were randomly assigned 1:1:1 to treatment with two different doses of bryostatin 1 (20 or 40 micrograms) or a placebo. The drug was to be administered via IV over 45 minutes. A total of seven doses were to be administered over 12 weeks.

The first dose for Mom was administered on January 15, 2016; the second on January 20; and the third on January 28. On February 23, after some testing was done, but before the infusion, we spoke with the doctor and decided to stop the trial. It was just too much for Mom to have to endure. She was experiencing some stomach pain and headaches. We did not know if this was related to the trial drug or not, but decided to stop the trial, just in case.

While I say that "we" decided to stop the trial, by this point in Mom's disease progression, she was unable to process information and make decisions for herself. She counted on me to make decisions for her. When asked a question, she would always look at me to respond for her. So, I was making this decision to stop the trial for my mom. Just like most decisions that I was now responsible for making for Mom, I questioned this one in my mind over and over again.

During the February 23 visit, Mom completed the MMSE-2 again. This time, her score was 8 out of 30. She could not answer the year, season, month, day of the week, date, or repeat three words after a pause. When asked to repeat, "It is a lovely, cool day but too windy," Mom said, "I can go outside with Terri. Too windy." When asked, "Got any plans for the weekend?" Mom said, "No.

At home. Not really. Terri comes with me and we do stuff together." When asked to write a sentence, what Mom wrote is shown in Figure 6.1 below.

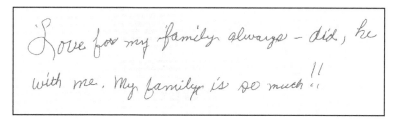

Figure 6.1.   The sentence Mom wrote on February 23, 2016.

When asked to draw intersecting pentagons (top picture shown in Figure 6.2), here is what Mom drew (bottom picture shown in Figure 6.2).

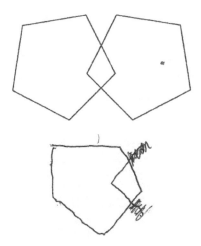

Figure 6.2.   Mom's drawing on February 23, 2016.

Reading back over my notes over three years later breaks my heart. It makes me question decisions I made. It makes me regret having put Mom through anything that was not 100% necessary at that stage in her disease. This is not to discount experimental trials or my belief in their importance. Without people willing or able to participate in trials, there is no chance for a cure or a method for controlling or reversing symptoms to be identified and brought to market for everyone's benefit. Dr. David Watson, founder of Alzheimer's Research and Treatment Center in Florida—which conducts clinical research for Alzheimer's disease—noted, "There is always a worse stage with this disease, associated with more loss and increased dependence. Trials can introduce hope for anyone at any stage."[1]

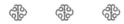

When you are considering the possibility of participating in a clinical trial for yourself or your loved one, there is a great deal of information that can help you understand the process and options, which may help you make your decisions.

The process of bringing a new drug to the market is long and costly, and it involves multiple public and private entities that fund and perform research and development. According to the United States Government Accountability Office (GAO) in its 2017 report on the drug industry, for "a new drug, the entire drug discovery, development, and review process can take up to 15 years, often accompanied by high costs."[2] The overall research and development process is shown below in Figure 6.3.

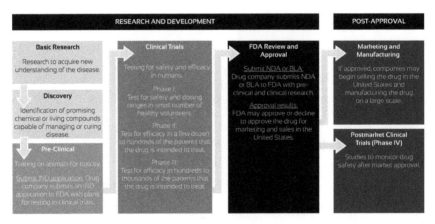

Figure 6.3. Stages in the typical brand name drug development process, from U.S. GAO 2017 report, *"Drug Industry: Profits, Research, and Development Spending and Merger and Acquisition Deals."*

The National Institutes of Health (NIH) listed 2,228 Alzheimer's disease studies in the database at www.clinicaltrials.gov at the time of this writing. The phase breakdown of these studies is shown in the pie chart in Figure 6.4.

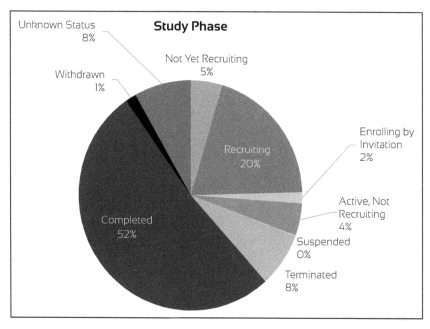

Figure 6.4. Data obtained from www.clinicaltrials.gov in November 2019. The total represented on this graph is 2,224. Study phase data was not provided for the remaining four studies.

More than half of the studies shown in the chart are already completed, and close to an additional quarter are done recruiting, have terminated, withdrawn, or are of unknown status. This leaves 580 studies that someone might consider for participation, including: 443 studies currently recruiting, 102 not yet recruiting, and 35 enrolling by invitation.

Of the 443 studies that are currently recruiting, 33 are identified as Phase III trials, listed in the Table 6.1 (the trials shown do not add up to 33, primarily due to some drugs involved in more than one trial and, thus, appearing in the database more than once). The clinical trials in Phase III are those that have made it through the rigor of two previous stages and are closest to opportunity for FDA approval (if Phase III is successful). This table relies on the www.clinicaltrials.gov database and shows what is in the drug development pipeline, recruiting at the time of this writing, and nearing the point of potential FDA approval (if there are clinical trial treatment options missing from this table, it is because, for some reason, they were not in the www.clinicaltrials.gov database or did not show up in the search process).

Table 6.1. Summary of Phase III trials recruiting in November 2019; data from www.clinicaltrials.gov

Drugs under study for Alzheimer's treatment	Icosapent ethyl (IPE); gantenerumab and solanezumab; azeilragon; ANVEX2-73; CAD106 and CNP520; gantenerumab alone; octohydroaminoacridine succinate; donepezil patch; AGB10; guanfacine with add-on therapy; BAN2401; TRx0237Angiotensin II receptor blocker (ARB, losartan) and calcium channel blocker (CCB, amlodipine) and atorivastatin
Drugs under study for a symptom associated with Alzheimer's	For insomnia: zolpidem and zoplicone For agitation: mirtazapine; brexipiprazole; AXS-05 and bupropion; AVP-786; COR388; escitalopram; For apathy: methylphenidate
Devices and behavioral interventions under study	Renew NCP-5; Amyloid PET#2; attention control condition and timed activity intervention; MRI and PET biomarkers; flutemetamol PET scanning
Dietary supplement interventions	Omega 3 treatment; Ginkgo biloba dispersible tablets;

Phase III can last for 30.5 months and approval can take six months to two years. Thus, even if the drugs and treatments shown here are successful in Phase III, it could take three to five more years before they are available for all patients.

The National Institutes of Health experimental trial database (www.clinicaltrials.gov) changes frequently, so it is important to visit the database to determine if there are any studies that may be of personal interest.

In addition, the TrialMatch® service offered by the Alzheimer's Association (https://trialmatch.alz.org/find-clinical-trials) allows anyone to input information about themselves or someone for whom they are a caregiver and receive a list of trials that may be a match for the specific circumstance. CenterWatch (http://www.centerwatch.com/clinical-trials/listings/) also provides a listing of clinical trials related to Alzheimer's disease. Their website identifies 614 clinical Alzheimer's trials at the time of this writing and allows a user to search by location for trials nearby. While the number of clinical trials posted on these websites seems promising, Dr. David Watson, as Principal Investigator on numerous trials for Alzheimer's disease himself, cautions that at any given time, there may be only one or two dozen Phase II or Phase III trials that represent strong clinical trial options for those impacted by Alzheimer's and dementia.[3]

As noted in previous chapters, much of the current experimental trial research is built upon the amyloid hypothesis, which is the assumption that accumulation of the peptide amyloid beta is the main cause of Alzheimer's disease. In recent years, though, the failures of several high-profile clinical trials of drugs targeting amyloid beta have provided a reason for researchers to explore alternative intervention targets.

One alternative theory is to attack both amyloid beta and tau simultaneously, despite the failure in 2016 of a phase III trial of a drug targeted as such. Inflammation is also seen as an important target. In the later stages of Alzheimer's disease, the immune cells of the brain, known as microglia, go into overdrive, killing neurons. Some researchers think that this is responsible for most symptoms of dementia, which means that inflammation could be a valuable target, even in people who are already experiencing symptoms.

Some researchers think that certain infections can cause Alzheimer's disease, which suggests that antimicrobial or antiviral drugs might have therapeutic value. They cite evidence showing that infection with herpes simplex virus (HSV), part of the human herpesvirus (HHV) family, influences a person's risk of Alzheimer's disease, and that variants of genes linked to sporadic Alzheimer's disease, such as APOE4, regulate immune function.

Earlier this year, a study in the journal *Neuron* revealed two strains of HHV (HHV-6A and HHV-7) that are more abundant in the brains of people with Alzheimer's disease.[4]

Another line of research is looking at the possibility of different types of amyloid beta structures and how these types might contribute to Alzheimer's disease. At the 2018 Alzheimer's Association International Conference (AAIC), an NIH researcher, Robert Tycko, PhD, senior investigator in the Laboratory of Chemical Physics, was honored for publication of "most impactful study of last two years." In this study, Tycko investigated the molecular structures of amyloid beta fibrils that develop in human brain tissue using solid-state nuclear magnetic resonance (ssNMR) to examine brain tissue and analyzed the possible associations between variations in these amyloid beta structures and how they might contribute to Alzheimer's disease.[5]

In addition to the newer research streams outlined above, there is currently a focus on research identifying additional biomarkers indicative of Alzheimer's disease beyond the use of spinal fluid testing and brain imaging. To aid in that research, Bill Gates announced in July 2018 that he joined a coalition of philanthropists who are investing $30 million to create a venture fund called Diagnostics Accelerator. In Gates's statement about the venture, he said, "We need a better way of diagnosing Alzheimer's—like a simple blood test or eye exam—before we're able to slow the progression of the disease ... Imagine a world where diagnosing Alzheimer's disease is as simple as getting your blood tested during your annual physical."[6] (More information about blood testing and retinal imaging for diagnosing Alzheimer's was presented in Chapter 2.)

Craig Ritchie, chair of the Psychiatry of Ageing at the University of Edinburgh and director of the Centre for Dementia Prevention, is one of the world's top authorities on clinical trials in dementia and has been the senior investigator on more than 30 drug trials. He's currently leading the PREVENT project, a study in the United Kingdom aiming to identify mid-life risks for dementia and to look at early changes in the brain. PREVENT is a prospective cohort study examining biomarker status at mid-life in at least 150 individuals genetically at high, medium, or low risk of late-onset Alzheimer's disease. Participants are children of individuals with or without a diagnosed Alzheimer's disease allocated to high-, medium-, and low-risk groups according to parental clinical status and APOE genotype. The biomarkers examined over two years include amyloid beta and tau levels in the plasma and cerebrospinal fluid.

Ritchie also leads the European Prevention of Alzheimer's Dementia Consortium (EPAD), which aims to build a network of trial delivery centers to carry out ongoing trials on prevention. EPAD is a public-private consortium, funded by the Innovative Medicines Initiative, designed to increase the likelihood of successful development of new treatments for the prevention of Alzheimer's dementia. EPAD will help with testing of different agents in this pre-dementia population through four components: improvement of access to existing cohorts and registries; development of the EPAD registry of approximately 24,000 people who might be at increased risk of developing Alzheimer's dementia; establishment of the EPAD Longitudinal Cohort Study of 6,000 people at any one time; and establishment of an adaptive proof-of-concept trial including 1,500 participants at any given time.

Last year, Ritchie wrote a paper called "The Edinburgh Consensus," which came out of a meeting of British experts in neurodegenerative diseases in Edinburgh.[7] The "consensus" was about the importance of identifying the disease in its early stages, since this is likely to be the time when treatments will work best. The key challenge, in terms of trials, he pointed out, was recruitment.

Successful recruitment into clinical trials is critical for the progression of research. Such research can lead to advancements in treatment overall and can also provide direct benefits to the people who participate. The decision to participate in clinical trials is, however, always up to each individual, their loved ones, and physicians.

What Next?

1. As early in the disease process as possible, start investigating the possibilities of clinical trial participation. Visit databases at the National Institutes of Health (www.clinicaltrials.gov), the Alzheimer's Association (https://trialmatch.alz.org/find-clinical-trials), and CenterWatch (http://www.centerwatch.com/clinical-trials/listings) to find trials that may be a match. Talk with your specialists about trials and opportunities they know of that could be beneficial.

2. Keep in mind that most trials in these databases are traditional drug-related trials. To find out more about novel or alternative approaches for Alzheimer's and dementias, read new books on the topic. You can find these simply by searching a website like www.amazon.com or www.bn.com for books on Alzheimer's and sorting by "newest to oldest" to find and order or pre-order books or asking a local bookstore to help you find them. Also, visit the Alzheimer's Association (https://www.alz.org) and Alzheimer's Disease International (https://www.alz.co.uk) websites often. Read the annual reports provided by each organization, and browse the sites for new updates of interest. In addition, the Alzheimer's Association International Conference website (https://www.alz.org/aaic/overview.asp) each year allows you to look for "highlights from the previous year," where you will find the newest research being discussed. Finally, visit websites such as www.alzheimersnewstoday.com, which provides up-to-date news on a range of topics related to Alzheimer's disease.

CHAPTER 7

CARE

> We both spent our entire lives wishing we could be something
> great. And now we're finally called upon to do something that
> requires some actual bravery, and you run and hide.
> —*From the movie,* **Wish I Was Here**

Mom did not want me to leave her during most of her illness, even during the early phase. While she was one of the most sociable people I knew before her illness, afterward, as the disease progressed, she felt most comfortable being with other people when she was with my brother, sister-in-law, or me.

There were clear signs of the disease progressing. For example, as the days and weeks passed, I could feel her trying so hard to hang on to her words, but slowly losing them. Conversations earlier in her disease sounded like this:

"I made cookies today," Mom said.

"You did. What kind of cookies?"

"Those ones with the little crunchy pieces. The light candies. You cut them in pieces and put them on a pan and cook them. And, they get bigger."

On another day, Mom said, "There is a big truck across the road. A lot of guys got out of it. They had machines. Big machines they ride on. They were cutting the grass."

I am longing to hang on to her words too. I listen closely and search for the things she is trying to say.

Mom's ability to express complete thoughts in a sentence was lost as her illness progressed, as was her ability to read or work on any kind of puzzle (she used to complete crosswords, for example). We began working on jigsaw puzzles together, and slowly over time, she could not see how the pieces fit together—even puzzles made for the youngest of children and even when I held the piece exactly where it was supposed to go. When the ability to have conversations, read, work on puzzles, cook, call friends, work on projects around the house, drive, run errands, and occupy yourself in any other way are gone, you depend completely on your loved ones/caregivers to help you occupy your time. What other option is there?

After my husband and I moved in with her, when I would try to sit at the desk and work in the home office, within minutes, Mom would make her way to the office and sit down in the chair in front of the desk. "When will you be done? How much longer do you have to work? What are you doing?" When her illness progressed a little further, more than a few times she asked, "Do you want to come and play?"

Every time Mom came and sat in that chair, I felt guilty, and I just wanted to get up and be with her. Usually, that was what I ended up doing.

Mom was slowly going to a different time and place in her mind. She would do things like talk to a child mannequin in an Old Navy store, thinking it was real. I also wondered why she paid such attention to certain things, such as jet streams in the sky, which she always pointed out. Or why, when we went on walks, she would always pick up small sticks, take them home, and put them in a stack in the garage. As many with Alzheimer's do, she also started to hide things, such as putting her coffee cup in her bedroom dresser drawer, and hiding her purse so well that there were many times that we traveled back to a store to see if she left it there.

Later in her illness when she would tell the story of riding in her father's truck, she would often look at me and ask, "Did you ever go with Daddy to sell his chickens?"

"No, I never got to," I would answer, knowing that she thought I was her older sister.

When we were out with new people, Mom would often tell them I was her mother, or her sister. For most of her illness, though, I was happy that she did remember my name, felt very comfortable with me, and knew I loved her.

When it got to the point that I realized I needed someone to spend time with Mom for a few hours here and there so I could run errands or try to work, I first reached out to one of Mom's church acquaintances and then to a family friend. These two women helped with Mom's care until they could no longer handle it. Mom had developed some habits that could be dangerous for Mom and for them.

Over time, Mom started to be terrified of being in a car and going some-place she did not want to go to. Even when coming home, Mom would get extremely upset and say, "This isn't the way home. You are going to run into the water! Stop it! Turn around!" She was convinced there was water ahead, and would reach for the door handle to try and open the door. This began to happen every time we would go anywhere and try to return home. It was so scary—not only for Mom but for her family members who were driving—that we began to avoid going anywhere. We never understood Mom's conviction that we were driving into the water. Perhaps it was related to a memory, or due to a halluci-nation, or something else entirely.

Family members were worrying more and more about Mom's safety. So, prompted by the beliefs of some of my other family members who, at the time, felt that we should at least try to find a place for Mom to live that could provide professional care for her around the clock, I took Mom to visit—or visited on my own or with my sister-in-law—three different live-in memory care places for Mom. I also took Mom to two different adult daycare places and dropped her off for their "trial day" to see how she liked it. When we went together to the live-in memory care centers, Mom was still able to look at me and say, "I'm not coming here. I'm not doing this."

The daycare centers were highly recommended, but sadly, I found them to be depressing. When I went to pick Mom up at one of them, I watched her through the door for a while without her knowing I was there. She was sitting among many others around a U-shaped table, while the person at the front of the room was trying to get everyone involved in an exercise of some sort. Mom was sitting there by herself, not interacting with the others in the room. When we left, I asked her about it. She said, "I don't want to go back." Truthfully, I did not blame her.

I say this fully aware that these options work wonderfully for some people. For us, though, even though I tried, I could never see having Mom go live anywhere but home with us. Even having her spend days in adult daycare centers did not feel right to me. I wanted her to have as much joy as she could each day and was convinced she needed to be with family to do that (even when she forgot who we were).

Our family did need more caregiving support though, so, in 2016, I began the process of working with caregiving agencies to have caregivers come to the home. We worked with three separate caregiving agencies and five separate caregivers over the course of about a year. Each agency was recommended by someone I knew and each agency said that their caregivers were experienced and trained in caring for someone with Alzheimer's and dementia. I learned over time that "experienced and trained" were relative terms, and should be discussed in much more depth with every caregiver a family considers hiring to help with their loved one. I also came to think that caring for someone with Alzheimer's and other dementia-related illnesses is very unique, and that it required a particular kind of caregiver—one not necessarily easily found.

In January 2016, we started working with the first caregiver. This caregiver was the worst experience of all. The caregiver called me once to have me talk to Mom to calm her down. Somehow the call got recorded in my voicemail, and I discovered it later that day. While there is more to the story, the caregiver was yelling at Mom and essentially threatening to take her to the hospital. Mom was terrified.

The second caregiver was not much better. Mom had started walking out of the front door. She was trying to go "home" I think, which, in her mind, was the house she grew up in. It was not until months later that I learned from a neighbor that when Mom would leave the house, the caregiver would go out in the driveway, sit in her car, listen to music, and watch Mom walk down the sidewalk until Mom came back on her own.

The third caregiver was a nice woman who loved to cook and spoiled us with her great meals. After working with Mom for about six weeks, she, however, let us know that she would have to quit. Mom was still walking out the front door. When she did, this caregiver followed her. But Mom had started to walk into the neighbors' homes. While these neighbors knew Mom, Mom still would go into their homes without knocking and surprise them. We were lucky that the neighbors, while quite agitated, understood enough to just talk to Mom, and that they were never surprised enough to do any harm to Mom. This caregiver quit after an instance when Mom walked all the way from her house to the front entrance of the neighborhood. The caregiver followed her and was able to get her to turn around and walk back home. The caregiver was so concerned about safety—for her and for Mom—that she quit. She really could not be blamed for that.

After this instance, I spoke with the owner of the home care agency, who was hesitant to place anyone else with Mom because of the wandering situation. She ended up agreeing to try again, and we installed a special lock on the front door so that Mom could not leave without assistance.

Unfortunately, though, Mom did not like the fourth caregiver at all, and because of this, I did not like leaving the house when she was there. Mom was still able to call me, and she did, typically minutes after I left. "Terri. Where are you? Can you come home? I'm here with this woman, and she's not very nice," she said. Once when I came home Mom had a scratch on her hand, which the caregiver proactively explained, saying that Mom hit her hand on the back of the bed. It did not look like that. It looked like someone scratched her, accidently or not.

At this time, I was leaving the house to run errands, to visit with a client for work, or to try and get work done elsewhere. I had my own consulting firm and much of my work could be done over the phone or on the computer, as long as I had a quiet space to do this. However, as time passed, I worked less and less, *and devoted more and more time to Mom. I did not feel comfortable leaving her with others who would let her walk out of the house and down the road. She would not do that when I was with her. I was fortunate that I had saved enough that I could live off of those savings for a while.*

When I think of these incidents, on the one hand, I feel guilt that I left Mom on her own with these caregivers, and did not know what was happening while I was gone. On the other hand, I had stayed at home with Mom and each of the caregivers for the first few weeks of each caregiver's employ to ensure that Mom was adjusting to the caregiver. Only after this initial adjustment period did I leave the house, leaving Mom and the caregiver alone. We also installed a few cameras in the house so I could check in during the day if I needed to be away.

Caring for Mom was becoming more challenging over time, of course. It was a 24-hour a day job, or as referenced in a famous book about Alzheimer's written by Nancy Mace, MA, and Peter Rabins, MD, a "36-hour day" job.[1] Not only did we install a new lock on the front door, and cameras in the house, but we also put a bed alarm on Mom's bed that would go off in my room if Mom tried to get out of bed or had an accident due to incontinence. It was typical for the alarm to go off almost every night, and for me to run to Mom's room to try to help her with whatever she needed, including getting to the bathroom, cleaning up if she was unable to get to the bathroom in time, or if she simply wanted to get out of bed.

In October, 2016, we found our next and final caregiver. She stayed with us until Mom's death, and was a godsend. On her first day, I was not sure if she would work out, as she followed Mom around the house, and I knew Mom did not like that. I talked with her about it and she quickly learned how to be more discreet in attending to Mom. More than anything else about her, you could tell she cared about Mom, and came to love Mom very quickly. She just had a loving, open, and caring spirit, and Mom could feel that. Mom loved her.

Although I did not know this would or could happen, she was my caregiver, too. She helped me on days when my knees buckled, and on days when I pretended to be strong.

In the last months, Mom responded better to her than to anyone else. When Mom would barely open her eyes, she would open them for this caregiver. When she would not eat for me or anyone else, she would eat for her.

We had found that one loving person who we needed to be with us and truly care for Mom for the remainder of her life.

 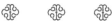

The role of caregiver is extremely difficult for a family member, even when—or perhaps because—there is so much love involved. The love for the family member going through Alzheimer's makes your heart break every day. You will mourn the loss of so many things along the way: the loss of their own life history and memories; the absence of friends and family members from their life; their ability to have a conversation with you or even say a word or two; the fact that they no longer know who you are exactly; their smile and laugh (they both go away in the end); the way that they used to love you so much and unconditionally—the list goes on.

Your loved one will have better days and worse days. Over the long term, you will try everything in your power to make sure they have what they need and as much joy as possible. That is your role—to watch over them and to make sure they are safe, never feel like a burden, and know that they are loved unconditionally. It goes back to that Hebrew word, *hesed* that author Lois Tverberg described as: "*hesed* acts out of unswerving loyalty … *hesed* is a love that can be counted on … It's not about the thrill of romance, but the security of faithfulness … *hesed* is not just a feeling but an action. It intervenes on behalf of loved ones and comes to their rescue."[2]

Many point to the increased difficulty of caring for a person with Alzheimer's or dementia due to the characteristics of the disease itself. While estimates vary, studies indicate that people age 65 and older survive an average of four to eight years after a diagnosis of Alzheimer's dementia, and some live as long as 20 years with Alzheimer's. This means that making care decisions can last for a decade or more for those in a family caregiver role. Individuals suffering with Alzheimer's disease also progress through many phases. Of the total number of years that they live with Alzheimer's dementia, individuals will spend an average of 40% of this time in dementia's most severe stage.[3] As the disease progresses, care needs change. Care choices may need to be re-evaluated again and again, and it is difficult to anticipate needs in a way that will minimize trauma and change for the person suffering with Alzheimer's. In addition, the loss of executive function associated with dementia can create hardships for caregivers in arranging care. Once the disease is too far progressed, the person with dementia can no longer participate in the long-term care planning process, so caregivers often have sole responsibility for life-altering decisions.

Long-term care is also very expensive and advanced financial planning is important to ensure a person suffering with Alzheimer's has the highest quality of care. Once the disease has progressed too far, the person will no longer be able to assist with decisions regarding paying for care. Finally, finding the right long-term care services for a loved one with Alzheimer's requires a lot of time, research, and energy. Meeting with several professionals or organizations to make any single service choice is not atypical. In addition, the loved one does not understand or cannot fully participate in the decision-making process.

The following sections provide information that may lessen some of the difficulties associated with maintaining care for a loved one.

Advanced Legal Planning

While it may not be intuitive to think of advanced planning as part of the care process, it can be one of the most critical steps in caring for a loved one with Alzheimer's. In some situations, the disease has already progressed so far that the person suffering with dementia can no longer do any planning. However, it can also happen that even when a family has indications that their loved one may be entering the disease process, they procrastinate talking with the person and helping to arrange important plans for a number of reasons. No one really wants to believe that this horrible disease may be coming. Everyone involved may try and deny it for as long as possible. That, of course, delays planning—perhaps to the point that the person with Alzheimer's can no longer make any decisions or be protected by some of the benefits that advanced planning can provide.

Several legal steps can be taken to clarify a person's wishes and ensure they have the right long-term support when they cannot make decisions themselves. During the legal planning process, a person's "legal capacity" may be considered, as it pertains to the ability to execute (put in place by signing) a legal document. Legal capacity is the ability to understand and appreciate the consequences of one's actions and to make rational decisions.

Legal capacity requirements can vary from one legal document to another. An elder law attorney can help determine what level of legal capacity is required for a person to sign a particular document. Creating a legal document does not imply that rights are immediately revoked. The legal forms that are completed will not be implemented until a person suffering with Alzheimer's or dementia legally no longer has the capacity to make decisions.

Consider completing the documents shown in Tables 7.1 and 7.2 (the information that follows is from the National Institute on Aging website):[4]

Table 7.1.   Advanced Healthcare Directives for People with Alzheimer's

Medical Document	How It Is Used
Living Will	Describes and instructs how the person wants end-of-life health care managed
Durable Power of Attorney for Health Care	Gives a designated person the authority to make healthcare decisions on behalf of the person with Alzheimer's
Do Not Resuscitate Order	Instructs healthcare professionals not to perform CPR in case of stopped heart or stopped breathing

Table 7.2. Advanced Directives for Financial and Estate Management

Legal/Financial Document	How It Is Used
Will	Indicates how a person's assets and estate will be distributed among beneficiaries after his/her death
Durable Power of Attorney for Finances	Gives a designated person the authority to make legal/financial decisions on behalf of the person with Alzheimer's
Living Trust	Gives a designated person (trustee) the authority to hold and distribute property and funds for the person with Alzheimer's

Advanced Insurance and Financial Planning

Long-term care can be very expensive. The AARP website (https://www.aarp.org/caregiving/financial-legal/info-2017/long-term-care-calculator.html) provides a long-term care calculator that lets people find the average costs for different types of services by state and metropolitan region, based on research by Genworth Financial. For example, in 2018, the most expensive option, a private room in a nursing home, costs $108,040 a year in a particular region of Florida. Assisted living facilities for those who cannot live independently but do not require skilled nursing care, cost about $42,450 a year in this region. For those seeking to remain at home, hiring a home health aide for 40 hours a week in the same region costs $47,840 a year. Other options include an adult day center, which charge an average of $70 a day or $27,040 a year for five days a week.

One research report found that the lifetime cost of care, including out-of-pocket costs, Medicare and Medicaid expenditures, and the value of informal caregiving, was $321,780 per person with Alzheimer's dementia in 2015 dollars ($341,840 in 2017 dollars).[5] Other researchers compared end-of-life costs for individuals with and without dementia. They found that the total cost in the last five years of life was $287,038 per person for individuals with dementia in 2010 dollars ($357,650 in 2018 dollars) and $183,001 per person for individuals without dementia ($228,020 in 2018 dollars), a difference of 57%. Out-of-pocket costs represented a substantially larger proportion of total wealth for those with dementia than for people without dementia (32% versus 11%).[6]

Given these high costs, it is important to consider how long-term care needs will be handled financially. Long-term care includes nonmedical care for people who have a chronic illness or disability and includes non-skilled personal care assistance (help with everyday activities, including dressing, bathing, toileting, adult day health care and other services).

Many people assume that Medicare in the United States will cover the costs associated with long-term care for a person with Alzheimer's and dementia. This is not the case. In general, Medicare and most health insurance plans, including Medicare Supplement insurance (Medigap) policies, do not pay for this type of care, sometimes called "custodial" care. The exception occurs when a person receives hospice services (to be discussed in Chapter 8), which are covered by Medicare insurance.

There is some confusion regarding this question of Medicare coverage for long-term care because Medicare is often mixed up with Medicaid. There are certain Medicare/Medicaid combination programs that cover some types of care, but a person with only Medicare insurance coverage will not receive care as a benefit.

While Medicare does not generally pay for home care or senior living, Medicaid does. By far, Medicaid's largest expenditures for the elderly are on long-term care. Given the high cost of care, many middle-income and even wealthy elderly Americans exhaust their assets, become "medically needy," and rely on Medicaid to pay the bills. As a result, over 60% of all nursing home residents are Medicaid beneficiaries. With respect to all long-term care services for the elderly, Medicaid is also the dominant payer, covering 45% of total costs.[7]

In order to participate in Medicaid, federal law requires states to cover certain groups of individuals. Low-income families, qualified pregnant women and children, and individuals receiving Supplemental Security

Income (SSI) are examples of mandatory eligibility groups. States have additional options for coverage and may choose to cover other groups, such as individuals receiving home- and community-based services and children in foster care who are not otherwise eligible.

The Affordable Care Act of 2010 created the opportunity for states to expand Medicaid. Under the Act, Medicaid eligibility would be extended to all individuals with incomes up to 133% of the federal poverty level beginning in 2014. Medicaid expansion would cover all families and individuals below this income level, including groups who are currently left out of public health coverage, such as low-income, able-bodied parents, low-income adults without children, and many low-income individuals with chronic mental illness or disabilities who struggle to maintain well-paid jobs but who do not currently meet disability standards for Medicaid.

The Supreme Court upheld the Affordable Care Act in 2012, but it gave the states the choice to opt out of Medicaid expansion. It now rests with governors and state legislatures to decide whether it is in the best interest of the state to implement the Medicaid portion of the law that affords health coverage to those in need. Visit https://www.healthinsurance.org/medicaid/ to find out if your state expanded its Medicaid coverage.

In addition, it is important to know that almost every state has multiple Medicaid programs. As a general rule of thumb, a person is eligible if: he or she has income and assets (not including a home and a car) less than 100 to 200% of the federal poverty level (FPL) and the person is pregnant, elderly, disabled, a parent/caretaker, or a child. If a person has income less than 133% of the FPL, there is possibly a program for him or her, depending on whether the state of residence expanded Medicaid coverage under the Affordable Care Act.

In 2018, the FPLs (in all states except Alaska and Hawaii, which have higher guidelines) are $12,140 with one person in the household; $16,460 with two people in the household; and $20,780 with three people in the household. When the state determines financial eligibility for Medicaid, it counts the following sources of income: regular benefit payments, such as

Social Security retirement or disability payments; veterans' benefits; pensions; salaries; wages; interest from bank accounts and certificates of deposit; and dividends from stocks and bonds. If Medicaid determines that you have given away or transferred your assets within the five years of the date you are applying (2.5 years in California), you will be ineligible for Medicaid benefits for a period of time. You are, however, allowed to transfer up to roughly $120,000 to your spouse if the spouse is not also applying for Medicaid and will continue to live independently.

In order to receive long-term care services under Medicaid, a medical specialist must document that Medicaid is needed through what is called "functional eligibility." Generally, a person must be unable to perform at least one of six activities of daily living on his or her own: bathing, dressing, using the toilet, transferring to or from a bed or chair, caring for incontinence, and eating.

If qualified, Medicaid will help pay for long-term care in a nursing home, skilled home health care services in a senior's private home, and short-term respite in a nursing home. It could also cover services to help stay at home, such as personal care and help with laundry and cleaning, according to the United States Department of Health and Human Services site, www.longtermcare.gov. Medicaid also pays for home renovations to keep people out of nursing homes, such as wheelchair ramps.

In addition to standard Medicaid options for care support, Medicaid waiver programs can also be considered. Under a Medicaid waiver, a state can waive certain Medicaid program requirements, allowing the state to provide care for people who might not otherwise be eligible under Medicaid. Through certain waivers, states can target services to people who need long-term service support. These waivers are called home- and community-based services (HCBS) 1915 waivers. Visit www.payingforseniorcare.com for state-specific waiver information and other information about paying for senior care.

HCBS waivers, issued by a state, can enable people who need significant services to stay out of institutional facilities and continue living at home.

HCBS provides no-cost care tailored to the individual, including assistance with daily living—such as homemaker services and personal care—and transportation to medical and therapy appointments.

To qualify, a person must be enrolled in Medicaid, fall within the resident's state income and asset criteria, meet the level-of-care and functional eligibility standards, and have a doctor-created plan of care. Benefits of this program depend on the state and may include home health aides, skilled nursing, personal care, hospice, case management, adult day services, adult day health care (offers nursing and therapy), transportation to medical care. meal programs, senior centers, friendly visitor programs, help with shopping and transportation, and help with legal questions, bill paying, or other financial matters.

Programs for All-Inclusive Care for the Elderly (PACE) is a Medicare and Medicaid-related program that helps people meet their health care needs in the community, instead of going to a nursing home or other care facility. PACE organizations provide care and services in the home, the community, and the PACE center. They have contracts with many specialists and other providers in the community to make sure that the care needed is provided. Many people in PACE get most of their care at the center from staff employed by the organization. PACE centers meet state and federal safety requirements. When enrolled in PACE, a person may be required to use a PACE-preferred doctor.

A person can have either Medicare or Medicaid, or both, to join PACE. PACE is only available in some states. The following qualifications exist for PACE: be 55 or older, live in the service area of a PACE organization (visit www.medicare.gov to search for PACE plans in the area), need a nursing home-level of care (as certified by your state), and be able to live safely in the community with help from PACE.

PACE provides all the care and services covered by Medicare and Medicaid, if authorized by the health care team. If a person's health care team decides that care and services are needed that Medicare and Medicaid do not cover, PACE may still cover them. Here are some of the services PACE covers: adult day primary care (including doctor and recreational therapy nursing services), dentistry, emergency services, home care, hospital care, laboratory/X-ray services, meals, medical specialty services, nursing home care, nutritional counseling, occupational therapy, physical therapy, prescription drugs, preventive care, social services (including caregiver training, support groups, and respite care), social work counseling, and transportation to the PACE center for activities or medical appointments, if medically necessary.

In addition to the health insurance coverage programs outlined above, do not overlook employer or union coverage, veteran's benefits, possible Medigap policy coverage (original Medicare's Supplemental Insurance), or long-term care insurance. Long-term care insurance can be especially important in easing the financial pains of a disease such as Alzheimer's.

Deciding on Long-Term Care Services

When the opportunity for advanced planning exists, it is important to have conversations about a loved one's feelings concerning various care options. The longer the conversation is postponed, the more difficult it will get. A person with Alzheimer's may develop paranoia and, if that happens, he or she may become suspicious of your efforts to discuss long-term care. He or she will also, of course, at some point, lose their capacity to provide any decision-making or input regarding their preferences.

While the average person who has never had a loved one with Alzheimer's may not know this, during the middle stages of Alzheimer's, it becomes necessary to provide 24-hour supervision to keep the person with dementia safe. In the late-stages, round-the-clock care requirements become more intensive. Consequently, it is important to realize that care choices may need to change over the course of the disease. Careful choices can lessen the long-term stress that an Alzheimer's afflicted person experiences.

Individuals may receive paid long-term care services in a variety of settings, including:

- in the community, such as at an adult day services center
- in the home, for example from a home health agency
- in institutions, such as in a nursing home
- in other residential settings, for instance in an assisted living or similar residential care community
- through hospice

In making decisions regarding long-term care services, different facets are important considerations, such as location, convenience, costs, meals and nutrition, and activities, as well as the stage of the disease. Perhaps most important, however, is the safety and well-being of a loved one. This has to do with the quality of care, which should be influenced in part by the level of regulation and inspection that exists for the different long-term care service options.

The Social Security Act mandates the establishment of minimum health and safety standards that must be met by providers and suppliers participating in the Medicare and Medicaid programs. These standards are found in the 42 Code of Federal Regulations—the principle set of rules and regulations issued by federal agencies of the United States regarding public health.

The Centers for Medicare and Medicaid Services (CMS) administers the standards compliance aspects of these programs. CMS develops Conditions of Participation (CoPs) and Conditions for Coverage (CfCs) that health care organizations must meet in order to begin and continue participating in the Medicare and Medicaid programs. There is a set of conditions for each type of provider or supplier subject to certification, found on the CMS website.[8] CMS also ensures that the standards of accrediting organizations recognized by CMS (through a process called "deeming") meet or exceed the Medicare standards set forth in the CoPs and CfCs.

For example, the CoPs for a Medicare-approved home health agency (HHA) require, among other things, that the HHA:[9]

- protect and promote the rights of each individual under its care;
- disclose ownership and management information required under HHA;
- not use as a home health aide (on a full-time, temporary, per diem, or other basis) any individual to provide items and services ... unless the individual has completed a training and competency evaluation program (CEP) or a CEP that meets minimum standards established ... and is competent to provide such items and services;
- operate and provide services in compliance with all applicable federal, state, and local laws and regulations

State Survey Agencies, under agreements between the state and the Secretary, carry out the Medicare certification process. The State Survey Agency is also authorized to set and enforce standards for Medicaid. State Survey Agencies perform initial surveys (inspections) and periodic resurveys (including complaint surveys) of all providers and certain kinds of suppliers. These surveys are conducted to ascertain whether a provider/supplier meets applicable requirements for participation in the Medicare and/or Medicaid programs and to evaluate performance and effectiveness in rendering a safe and acceptable quality of care. After the State Survey Agency completes an inspection for the Medicare/Medicaid program, it submits evidence and a certification recommendation for a final CMS Regional Office determination.

To find the State Survey Agency that services a particular state, visit the Association of Health Facilities Survey Agencies at www.asfsa.org and click on "AHFSA State Agency Sites." For example, in Florida, the regulating agency is the Agency for Health Care Administration (AHCA). Visiting the regulating agency website (www.ahca.myflorida.com in this case) generally provides more information about the specific state regulations involved, as well as a listing of all the adult day centers for the state and by account, along with the licensure number when available. In Florida, the AHCA also provides a service at www.floridahealthfinder.gov that allows the user to search for facilities of any type and locate detailed information about inspections and results.

The following section provides more information on each of the long-term care service options and any regulation that occurs beyond the Medicare and/or Medicaid certification.

Adult Day Services Centers

Adult day services centers offer people with Alzheimer's and other dementias the opportunity to be social and to participate in activities in a safe environment. A number of options are available in almost any community, and they vary in the services provided and the rates, so calling and visiting local centers is important. Transportation to and from the center is often provided. Many centers also offer a complementary trial day for the person needing care. Trying this option earlier in the disease may make it easier for the person with dementia to adjust and begin new relationships.

Adult daycare is generally divided into two types, adult day services and adult day health services. Adult day services include supervised activities, meals, socialization, and limited health services. Adult day health services provide structured therapeutic health services and supervised activities for people with physical, mental, or intellectual disabilities or the aged who meet nursing facility level-of-care requirements. The largest percentage of adult day centers are equally social and medical (40%) and 31% are primarily social with some medical.[10]

The Centers for Disease Control and Prevention (CDC) also reports that the top ten diseases represented among users of adult day services are, in order, hypertension, arthritis, diabetes, Alzheimer's disease or other dementias (31%), depression, heart disease, osteoporosis, chronic obstructive pulmonary disease, asthma, and chronic kidney disease. Overall, 69%

of adult day service programs offer specific programs for individuals with Alzheimer's or other dementias, and 14% of adult day service centers primarily serve individuals with Alzheimer's or other dementias.[11]

Genworth provides a survey of cost of care information on a yearly, monthly, daily, and hourly basis for in-home care (homemaker services and home health aides), community and assisted living (adult day health care and assisted living facility), and nursing home facility (semi-private room and private room). Median cost of care is provided for each kind of care for the United States nationally and for each state in the United States. While the survey does not cover every type of service, it gives people a resource where they can begin with a strong estimate of what services will cost. For the 2019 survey, the median cost of adult day health care for the United States nationally was $19,500 per year or $1,625 per month or $75 per day.[12]

As noted, state Medicaid waiver programs approved by CMS may pay for adult day services or adult day health services provided according to a person-centered plan of care, for beneficiaries who meet nursing facility or institutional level-of-care requirements or are at risk of institutionalization.

The approach to regulation of adult day services centers varies widely by state. The majority of states regulate adult day service through certification and/or licensure. It is important to look at the requirements of a specific state to determine what exactly these concepts mean, as for at least three states, there are no differences between them, and certification is equivalent to licensure. In general, though, those services wishing to receive reimbursement from Medicare and/or Medicaid must also be certified by the state. Some states require both certification and licensure, and some require neither.

Table 7.3 provides a summary of state requirements of adult day services as of the United States Department of Health and Human Services's last regulatory review of adult day services in 2014.[13]

Twenty-five states have specific requirements for providers that serve people with dementia: Alaska, Arkansas, California, Delaware, Florida, Georgia, Iowa, Kansas, Kentucky, Louisiana, Maine, Massachusetts, Michigan, Minnesota, Missouri, Nevada, New Hampshire, New Jersey,

Table 7.3. State Requirements for Adult Day Services

State	Licensure Only	Certification Only	Licensure + Certification	Other Requirements
Alabama				X
Alaska		X		
Arizona	X			
Arkansas	X			
California			X	
Colorado		X		
Connecticut		X		
Delaware	X			
District of Columbia				X
Florida	X			
Georgia	X			X
Hawaii	X			
Idaho				X
Illinois		X		
Indiana				X
Iowa		X		
Kansas	X			
Kentucky			X	
Louisiana	X			
Maine	X			
Maryland			X	
Massachusetts	X			X
Michigan				X
Minnesota	X			
Mississippi				X

(continued)

Table 7.3. State Requirements for Adult Day Services *(continued)*

State	Licensure Only	Certification Only	Licensure + Certification	Other Requirements
Missouri	X			
Montana	X			
Nebraska	X			
Nevada			X	X
New Hampshire	X			
New Jersey	X			X
New Mexico	X			
New York				X
North Carolina		X		
North Dakota				X
Ohio		X		
Oklahoma	X			
Oregon		X		X
Pennsylvania	X			
Rhode Island	X			
South Carolina	X			
South Dakota				X
Tennessee	X			
Texas	X			
Utah	X			
Vermont		X		
Virginia	X			
Washington				X
West Virginia	X			
Wisconsin		X		
Wyoming	X			

North Carolina, Pennsylvania, Rhode Island, South Dakota, Tennessee, Utah, and West Virginia.

States' requirements may apply to any adult day services program that serves people with dementia or only to programs that exclusively serve this population. Any additional requirements generally relate to staffing and training, such as requiring lower staff-to-participant ratios and dementia-specific training for all staff. The Justice in Aging organization (www.just iceinaging.org) provides an excellent 2015 summary of dementia-specific training requirements for every state and every professional license category in a report titled, "Training to Serve People with Dementia: Is our Health-care System Ready?" which can be found on the website.[14]

In considering adult daycare options, it is important to understand a particular state's regulation process and, at a minimum, ensure that a provider being considered meets this process. A good place to find this information is the State Survey Agency for a specific state. The State Survey Agencies are provided at the following site: https://www.cms.gov/Medi-care/Provider-Enrollment-and-Certification/SurveyCertificationGenInfo/Downloads/Survey-and-Certification-State-Agency-Contacts.pdf. Doing so for Florida, as an example, provides a link for finding a facility, which connects to https://www.floridahealthfinder.gov/facilitylocator/FacilitySearch.aspx and allows for searching for a particular type of facility by state or area. This yields a full list of agencies and allows for clicking on a particular agency for information about that agency. For Florida, a list of 340 active adult daycare centers, including the license number and type, license expiration date, owner, and contact information can also be found here: (https://ahca.myflorida.com/MCHQ/Health_Facility_Regulation/Assisted_Living/docs/adcc/Directory_ADCC_11.04.19.pdf).

Home Care Agencies

Home care agencies provide services in the home, rather than in a hospital or care facility. The service can allow a person with Alzheimer's or other dementia to stay in his or her own home. It also can be of great assistance to family caregivers. In general, there are two types of home care agencies: a medical skilled home health agency and a nonmedical home care agency. Both can include companion services (help with supervision, recreational activities, or visiting), personal care services (help with bathing, dressing, toileting, eating, exercising, or other personal care), and homemaker services (help with housekeeping, shopping, or meal preparation). Only a medical skilled home health agency can provide help with medical needs (e.g., wound care, injections, and physical therapy) by a licensed health professional. Home health care is medical and prescribed by a doctor, but home care is nonmedical and does not require a doctor's prescription. Unless there is a short-term distinct medical need for a person with Alzheimer's or other dementia that is ordered by a doctor, typically, long-term care provided for people with Alzheimer's and other dementias is provided by nonmedical home care agencies.

Every state except for Idaho, South Dakota, and Vermont requires home health agencies to go through some type of certification. Agencies providing any services covered by Medicare must be certified and monitored by the U.S. Department of Health and Human Services's Centers for Medicare and Medicaid Services. For nonmedical home care agencies, far fewer states have certification requirements.

Each State's Survey Agency provides more complete information about home care providers. Just as with adult day centers, in Florida, for example, visiting https://www.floridahealthfinder.gov/facilitylocator/FacilitySearch.aspx and searching for either "Home Health Agency" for home health agencies or "Homemaker and Companion Services" for nonmedical home care service agencies provides a list of agencies of either type (the search can be narrowed down to focus on a particular region or a particular agency as well). Clicking on a particular agency provides information about that agency, including license number, license term, inspection reports and details, and any emergency actions.

In addition, for home health agencies, visiting the following website allows for a direct comparison of agencies in a state or particular region: https://www.medicare.gov/homehealthcompare/search.html. Quality of patient care ratings, including ratings provided through patient surveys, are provided here and allow for a more direct comparison of facilities.

Because nonmedical home care agencies do not have the same licensure or certification requirements as home health agencies, it can be more difficult to determine what quality standards are sure to exist for these agencies. When seeking this kind of care, people who have Alzheimer's and their loved ones often need to rely on more anecdotal evidence, such as referrals from people they know.

In terms of the costs associated with home care, Alzheimer's care at home can be more affordable than residential care. Typically, home care providers do not charge additional fees to care for individuals with Alzheimer's. This is not the case in senior living residences where Alzheimer's and dementia care usually costs an additional $1,200 per month.

Both home care aides and home health aides bill on an hourly basis (with the exception of live-in caregivers, who sometimes bill flat rates). Home care aides can be retained through a home care agency or by hiring private caregivers. Home health aides experience greater federal regulation and are almost always hired through an agency. Home health aides visit the home as much as medically necessary; typically for shorter periods of time than home care aides.

The median cost in the United States for a paid nonmedical home aide is $51,480 per year, $4,290 per month, $141 per day, and $22.50 per hour. For a medical home health aide, the median costs are $52,624 per year, $4,385 per month, $144 per day, and $23 per hour.[15] Private individuals can be retained to provide most of the same services with fees that are 20 to 30% lower. However, independent caregivers are typically uninsured, do not go through background checks, and may be unable to provide backups if they are not available to work on short notice.

Nursing Homes

In 2014, 50% of nursing home residents had Alzheimer's or other dementias.[16]

Nursing home admission by age 80 is expected for 75% of people with Alzheimer's dementia compared with only 4% of the general population.[17]

The median cost for a private room in a nursing home in the United States is $102,200 per year, $8,517 per month, and $280 per day; the median cost for a semiprivate room is $90,155 per year, $7,513 per month, and $247 per day.[18]

Nursing homes are almost always Medicare and Medicaid certified. Nursing homes that receive funds from Medicare or Medicaid must comply with federal regulations established in the 1987 Nursing Home Reform Act and subsequent updates.

In 1987, President Ronald Reagan signed into law the first major revision of the federal standards for nursing home care since 1965. The landmark legislation changed society's legal expectations of nursing homes and their care. Long-term care facilities wanting Medicare or Medicaid funding were to provide services so that each resident can attain and maintain her highest practicable physical, mental, and psychosocial well-being.

The Federal Nursing Home Reform Act created a set of national minimum standards of care and rights for people living in certified nursing facilities. Some of the most important resident provisions include:[19]

- emphasis on a resident's quality of life as well as the quality of care;
- new expectations that each resident's ability to walk, bathe, and perform other activities of daily living will be maintained or improved absent medical reasons;
- a resident assessment process leading to development of an individualized care plan;
- 75 hours of training and testing of paraprofessional staff;

- rights to remain in the nursing home absent nonpayment, dangerous resident behaviors, or significant changes in a resident's medical condition;
- uniform certification standards for Medicare and Medicaid homes; and
- prohibitions on turning to family members to pay for Medicare and Medicaid services

In 2016, CMS further revised the requirements that long-term care facilities must meet to participate in the Medicare and Medicaid programs. The new regulations were effective November 28, 2016, and included phases to be implemented over the next several years. The complete document outlining updates can be found at www.federalregister.gov.[20]

The CMS provides Nursing Home Compare as a web-based report card, available at https://www.medicare.gov/nursinghomecompare/search. html. Using a five-star rating, the agency assesses the quality of care of CMS-certified nursing homes. By typing in a zip code, one is able to see an overall ratings and ratings on health inspections, staffing, and quality measures of nursing homes in the area. The site always allows for the comparison of up to three nursing homes, providing in-depth information about the inspections and ratings of each. While an excellent resource, Nursing Home Compare does not evaluate assisted living or senior housing options not funded by Medicare.

In addition to Medicare and Medicaid certifications and regulations in all states, as well as the District of Columbia, long-term care/nursing home administrators are required to possess a state license, which generally involves completing an accredited, state-approved training program (usually a bachelor's degree), completing an internship, and passing a state/national licensing examination. Most states use the National Association of Long-Term Care Administrator Boards (NAB) Nursing Home Administrator Exam (NHA) for licensure. Some states also use a state examination.

Residential Care Communities and Assisted Living

An assisted living residence is a long-term senior care option that, in general, provides basic medical monitoring and help with activities of daily living (ADLs) such as dressing, eating, mobility, hygiene, bathing, toileting, using the telephone, and shopping. Since each state and province have different licensing and regulation requirements for assisted living providers, the particular services offered varies. For example, some assisted living facilities are attached to or share a campus with a skilled nursing facility. This means these types of communities can provide more advanced medical care.

Memory care units (also called Alzheimer's Special Care Units or SCUs) often exist as part of another facility, such as a nursing home. Continuing care retirement communities (CCRCs) provide different levels of care—independent, assisted living, and nursing home. Based on individual needs, a resident is able to move throughout the different levels of care within the community if his or her needs change.

The median cost for care for a private, one-bedroom quarters in an assisted living facility in the United States is $48,612 per year, $4,051 per month, and $133 per day.[21]

According to the CDC, 40% of residents in residential care facilities, including assisted living facilities, have Alzheimer's or other dementias. Small residential care facilities (4 to 25 beds) have a larger proportion of residents with Alzheimer's or other dementias than larger facilities (47% in facilities with 4 to 25 beds compared with 42% in facilities with 26 to 50 beds and 37% in facilities with more than 50 beds). More than half (58%) of residential care facilities offer programs for residents with Alzheimer's or other dementias.

Assisted living facilities are not Medicare certified; 48% are Medicaid certified. Assisted living facilities are mostly paid for privately, but some do accept Medicaid. In general, assisted living facilities and senior housing are regulated by the states. Each state issues a license to a facility after an inspection, typically conducted annually or semiannually. This process is overseen by a state's Department of Health, Department of Social Services, or, in some instances, a combination of these departments. Inspection teams typically comprise nurses, social workers, sanitarians, and public health officials. The teams survey staff, residents, and family members; examine facility records; and make observations. These surveys are then used to identify compliance and quality improvement issues.

Most state regulations address essential services that a senior living facility must provide. These services include assistance with ADLs. Some states have additional regulations for services, such as money management, making medical appointments, and taking residents shopping. Keep in mind that many senior housing communities that provide only housing, housekeeping, and meals are not required to be licensed by the states.

Most states also do not license residential care/assisted living administrators. A few states that require licensure, including South Carolina and Virginia, require candidates for licensure to possess an associate's degree. Hawaii is the only state to require a bachelor's degree for residential care/assisting living administration licensure.

Unpaid or Family Caregivers

Of course, in addition to the professional paid services outlined above, unpaid (usually family) caregivers provide the primary care in many situations. The Alzheimer's Association "2018 Alzheimer's Disease Facts and Figures" report notes that there are 16.1 million Americans who provide unpaid care for people with Alzheimer's or other dementias. These caregivers provide an estimated 18.4 billion hours of care valued at over $232 billion.[22]

Unpaid caregivers spend countless hours with the people they care for, sometimes with little support from others, despite being a critical component of their community and society. The 2017 Carers Report: "Embracing the Critical Role of Caregivers Around the World," published by Merck KGaA, notes:[23]

- Almost 3 in 10 (28%) of unpaid caregivers feel their role as a caregiver is unrecognized by their health care system.
- Approximately 43% of unpaid caregivers who live in suburban areas do not feel supported at all in their role as an unpaid caregiver by social/ welfare services.
- 57% of female unpaid caregivers do not feel supported at all in their role as an unpaid caregiver by the government.

Much research supports the unique nature of caring for a person with Alzheimer's. Care can last for several years, as the duration of the disease is long. Care can be very intimate and even intrusive. For example, care often includes help with bathing, toileting, and incontinence. The emotional and mental stress experienced by a caregiver can be tremendous. Caregivers are often on call around-the-clock for someone who perhaps does not even know who they are anymore. At a certain stage, care may also involve physical demands on the caregiver required to transfer their loved one to bed or to a toilet, for example. The emotional, mental, and physical demands can lead to health problems for the caregiver. In addition, caring for a loved one can have a negative effect on employment, income, and financial security. Caregivers may need to go from working full time to part time, take leaves of absence, or even quit work entirely.

Person- and Relational-Centered Care

Chapter 4 provided information about person- and relational-centered care for people with Alzheimer's and other dementias. As noted in that chapter, the Alzheimer's Association published its 2018 Dementia Care Practice Recommendations, with person-centered care at the foundation of these recommendations. As previously noted, the following practice recommendations are at the core of person-centered care:

1. Know the person living with dementia.
2. Recognize and accept the person's reality.
3. Identify and support ongoing opportunities for meaningful engagement.
4. Build and nurture authentic, caring relationships.
5. Create and maintain a supportive community for individuals, families, and staff.
6. Evaluate care practices regularly and make appropriate changes.

International Stage and the Role of Community in Dementia Care

Dementia has been the focus of increased global collaboration and discussion, beginning with the G8 Dementia Summit in London in December 2013, which formed the World Dementia Council. The first Ministerial Conference on Global Action Against Dementia, organized by the World Health Organization (WHO), and supported by the Organization of Economic Cooperation and Development (OECD), took place in March 2015. The OECD is a forum where governments work together to address the economic, social, and environmental challenges of globalization. The OECD member countries are: Australia, Austria, Belgium, Canada, Chile, Czech Republic, Denmark, Estonia, Finland, France, Germany, Greece, Hungary, Iceland, Ireland, Israel, Italy, Japan, Korea, Luxembourg, Mexico, the Netherlands, New Zealand, Norway, Poland, Portugal, the Slovak Republic, Slovenia, Spain, Sweden, Switzerland, Turkey, the United Kingdom, and the United States.

As an outgrowth of these efforts, WHO published the "Global action plan on the public health response to dementia 2017–2025," which was adopted in May 2017 and includes seven targets for improved policy, awareness, risk reduction, diagnosis and treatment, carer support, information systems, and research.[24] The first target, "Dementia as a public health priority," urges that 75% of Member States (146 countries) must develop a tailored response to dementia by 2025. The U.S. plan was updated in 2019 and called the "National Plan to Address Alzheimer's Disease: 2019 Update." Other countries with a national plan include: Australia, Austria, Chile, Costa Rica, Cuba, Czech Republic, Denmark, Finland, France, Greece, Indonesia, Ireland, Israel, Italy, Japan, Korea, Luxembourg, Malta, Mexico, Netherlands, Norway, Slovenia, Switzerland, and the United Kingdom.

One of the indicators for improvement of the WHO objective of improving awareness is "dementia-friendly initiatives." According to WHO, key aspects of dementia-friendly initiatives include safeguarding the human rights of people with dementia, tackling the stigmatization associated with dementia, promoting a greater involvement of people with dementia in society, and supporting families and carers of people with dementia.

A good example of dementia-friendly initiatives is the creation of Memory Cafes. With roots in the Netherlands, Dr. Bere Miesen, a Dutch psychiatrist, introduced the Memory Cafe concept in 1997 as a way to break through the stigma associated with various forms of dementia. The concept spread throughout Europe, Australia, and eventually to the United States. Today, hundreds of Memory Cafes take place in a wide range of venues on a regular basis in the United States. You can choose to visit more than one. When regional Cafe operators vary their schedules, you are able to attend several of them on a rotating basis. Visit www.memorycafedirectory to find gatherings near you.

Dementia-friendly communities are a natural extension of dementia-friendly initiatives. Alzheimer's Disease International (ADI) defines a dementia-friendly community as a place or culture in which people with dementia and their carers are empowered, supported, and included in society, understand their rights, and recognize their full potential.

Dementia-friendly communities have as their end goal a better life for people with dementia. ADI suggests that the four essential elements needed to support a dementia-friendly community are people, communities, organizations, and partnerships.[25] More specifically, dementia-friendly communities should be shaped around the needs and opinions of people living with dementia and their caregivers. Communities need to tackle the stigma and social isolation associated with dementia and ensure that physical environments support people with dementia. Encouraging organizations to establish dementia-friendly approaches and implement strategies that help people with dementia will contribute to a dementia-friendly society. Finally, working in collaboration and partnership is critical to dementia-friendly communities. ADI provides a summary of dementia-friendly communities established in a number of countries around the world.

ACT on Alzheimer's was established in June 2011 as a state-wide initiative to make Minnesota more dementia friendly. The Dementia Friendly America (DFA) initiative was launched in the United States in 2015 based on ACT on Alzheimer's, a model initiative from the state of Minnesota. DFA is a national cross-sector effort to help communities better understand, embrace, and support residents living with dementia. To help communities work toward becoming dementia friendly, DFA offers technical assistance, including a community tool kit, sector-specific guidance, and best practices synthesized from across the world. For these resources and to learn how to join the DFA network of communities, visit www.dfamerica.org.

In 2009, the first kind of residential dementia village appeared in Hogeweyk, Holland, outside Amsterdam. Inhabitants walk freely among the walled town's parklike grounds and live in housing units arranged by theme. There are also grocery stores, hair salons, and pubs where the staff works and keeps an eye on the 152 residents. The village is about the size of ten football fields.

In the United States, there are some that are taking similar approaches to those described above, although not identical. Grassroots organizations and initiatives have developed to support and advance dementia-friendly initiatives and communities. For example, Dementia-Friendly Communities of Northern Colorado, founded by Cyndy Luzinski, was launched in 2015, for this reason.

Prairie Elder Care in Kansas has a dementia-care residence farm in Overland Park, Kansas called Prairie Farmstead. It has chicken coops and gardens. It can accommodate about 16 residents, who will always be supervised, and they can also plant tomatoes or roam in a sensory garden with butterflies.

Scott Tarde, chief executive officer of George G. Glenner Alzheimer's Family Centers, has launched a faux mini-town (town within a building) with a 1950s and 1960s look designed for people with dementia: Glenner Town Square. His concept is based on reminiscence therapy. Tarde wants to build 100 of these daycare centers throughout the United States within 20 years. To be sure, a "faux" town is not the same as the concept first implemented in Holland.

While there remains so much to be done to realize the vision of being dementia friendly, for communities and for individuals, with careful thought, planning, and creativity, caregivers can find or create environments in the home and community that provide the person-centered care their loved one deserves.

What Next?

1. No matter what your health situation, any adult needs to ensure that they have all appropriate legal papers completed, for their benefit and for the benefit of their loved ones. Even when all legal documents are completed, there will still be significant issues or topics for a loved one to work through, because everything has not been anticipated or because of the paperwork involved after a person's death. If you are caring for someone who has Alzheimer's or dementia and they have not completed needed legal documents, help them achieve this as soon after diagnosis as you can. Make sure all children are involved in this process, if possible. This will avoid later confusion, misunderstandings,

or disagreements. Avoid concerns regarding "legal capacity" by working with an elder law attorney and taking this step as early as possible, and videotaping capacity assessments made by these attorneys.

2. Paying for Alzheimer's and dementia care is very expensive. Even if you intend to provide unpaid family care for the duration of the disease, there is much that can go wrong with this plan. If a person has almost no financial resources, Medicaid will support much of the financial care burden. However, the quality of care may be variable. Make sure to consider the various scenarios and options available to help ensure that care resources can be provided, and that the financial burden is as minimal as necessary.

3. Stay informed about legislation that can assist with care needs for those with Alzheimer's and dementia and the needs of caregivers themselves. You might do this by setting up a Google alert for "Alzheimer's legislation," for example. (Google alerts can easily be set up for any topic by going to www.google.com/alerts). Get behind or in front of legislation that you see as critical in this regard. The United States may be behind other countries in terms of support for care, allowing for care concerns to be placed on the backs of many family members who take on costs of care themselves, while also needing to quit jobs to provide care, but the voices of those affected by the disease can make a difference.

4. Use the information provided in this chapter to look up costs, ratings, certifications, etc. for the various care options you are considering. Call and visit options that look most viable in advance of the need. Take your loved one to visit options. Watch how people interact with them and pay attention to their expressed or unexpressed needs and desires.

5. If you decide to provide unpaid family care for your loved one, go into it as fully prepared and aware as possible. Early in the disease, try to have open family conversations about how various family members can best support the process (almost like role negotiations). If a family member lives in another state and cannot be there physically to support the

process as much as desired, perhaps they can provide some additional financial support. Try to firm up commitments early, because later, as the disease progresses, everyone will be under so much stress that rational discussions are less possible.

6. If you do decide to provide care for your loved one and your loved one has the resources to pay you, just as they would for professional help, consider establishing a legal arrangement to make this possible. While many people feel guilty about doing this (as I did and therefore, I did not do it, even though both my mother and her attorney suggested it), if you need to stop working to care for a family member, you may not only lose income, but also lose all of your savings just to pay for ongoing expenses. Your loved one would not want that to happen. Let family members know in advance that this is happening.

7. Trust your instincts about the people and organizations providing care for your loved one. You should feel that they truly care about your loved one. It is not too much to ask that you feel that they even have love for your loved one. You will find the person who does care for and love your loved one if you trust your instincts and judgment and keep looking.

8. Implement several practical tools for the safety, security, and well-being of your loved one. For example, purchase a bed alarm that allows you to know when you loved one is getting out of bed or when they have had an accident related to incontinence. Install door locks or alarm systems so you know that your loved one cannot go outside without someone being aware of it. Purchase systems that provide tracking or warning if they wander, despite all efforts to avoid it. Consider installing nanny cams in your home if you have any concerns about what happens when you need to be away. While many of these ideas are learned over time with experience, the NIA website provides a good starting list for ensuring the safety of those with Alzheimer's (https://www.nia.nih.gov/health/home-safety-checklist-alzheimers-disease).

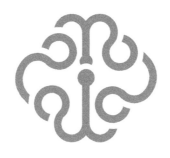

PART THREE

"GIVE IT TO GOD."

The End of Life with Alzheimer's Disease

CHAPTER 8

HOSPICE

The truth is that there is only one terminal dignity—love. And the story of a love is not important—what is important is that one is capable of love. It is perhaps the only glimpse we are permitted of eternity.
—*Helen Hayes*

Mom was admitted into the in-home hospice program (Trustbridge in our case) on October 20, 2016.

This decision happened after asking Mom's general practitioner whether he thought this was a direction we should consider at that time. This general practitioner was another person in our life at the time who I trusted completely. He cared for Mom. She cared for him. He always offered sound and compassionate advice.

At this juncture, he thought that referring Mom to hospice was appropriate. He also discussed the potential benefits of hospice care with us, as well as things that we should know. As I remember it, he let us know that hospice is generally considered as an option in the last six months of life. Once admitted, Mom would be re-evaluated at key junctures (such as the six-month point) to determine if hospice care was still appropriate. In some patient situations, some recovery happens and the person might exit the program for a while, perhaps returning later. He also let us know that once hospice was involved, that the hospice medical team really took the lead regarding any major medical advice. Mom would still see him as we needed or wanted, but the hospice doctor essentially became the doctor in charge of Mom's care.

Once Mom was in hospice, there would be a set team of people who came to the house on a fairly regular basis to watch over and care for her. This support was covered by Medicare. In addition, anything Mom needed in terms of supplies, medications, equipment, etc. would be ordered by the team and be delivered to our home.

It seemed like the right decision to make for Mom, and I am glad I did make it. The hospice team was a wonderful support for Mom and for me.

On the day Mom was admitted into the program, a member of the hospice team recorded the following notes (all notes taken by hospice and hospital staff in this chapter are provided as transcribed, with the exception that the names of professionals are excluded). The hospice doctor made his first visit a few weeks later and made notes to Mom's file.

October 20, 2016

Patient lives with her daughter Terri. Has private aide 3 times a week. Patient has been declining last several months with increasing weakness, decreased appetite, weight loss, increasing confusion, incontinence, tremors, rare pain in both shoulders, falls, some diarrhea. Patient is disoriented to time and place. FAST 7a. PPS 40. BMI 21. Sleeps approximately 15 hours a day. Daughter's goal is to keep patient home with comfort care. DNR discussed but not signed today as daughter needs to find advanced directives to see what they say. Daughter states she is health care surrogate. Will admit today.

November 2, 2016

77-year-old female with a diagnosis of senile degeneration of the brain. The patient is sitting at the kitchen table and eating lunch. She is able to feed

---

> *herself. She does say several words but cannot answer my simple questions. Her speech often drifts into gibberish. The history is obtained from the patient's family. The family informs me that the patient does complain of pain at both shoulders and both arms. The patient is unable to describe the pain. She is unable to rate the pain. The family will administer Tylenol with good relief. The family reports that the patient will complain of pain when she is being transferred to a bed and requires some assistance. The family also reports that the patient has a poor appetite. One year ago the patient weighed 154. She has lost more than 10% of her weight and now weighs 124. Her BMI is 22. The patient is weak. With help, the patient can stand up.*

Some of the notations in Mom's medical records were new to me. The BMI, as most people know, is Body Mass Index. The FAST notation refers to the Functional Assessment Staging Test used to determine current stage of the disease. When admitted into hospice, this stage was determined to be 7a for Mom (the FAST stages are shown in Chapter 3). The PPS level notation refers to Palliative Performance Scale. No one ever told me about PPS assessment when Mom was in hospice, although it would have helped me to better understand Mom's condition. Mom's PPS the day she was admitted to hospice was 40%. Table 8.1 shows the PPS levels and interpretation.

A few weeks after the doctor's visit, we encountered a setback we did not expect. I went to wake Mom up in the morning, and she could not step down on her foot. I knew she had not gotten out of bed in the night and hurt it because we had an alarm on the bed that would go off in my room when Mom got up. It never went off. But, somehow, she either hurt her ankle the day before or twisted it in bed at night. I called 911.

The ER did a number of tests but found nothing significant and gave the discharge orders. Mom, however, had not improved at all and was unable to put any weight on her foot. She also was so far along in her disease and confused at the time and could not really assist in her own movement. This was one of those times when the interplay between hospice and the ER staff was very frustrating.

Table 8.1.   Palliative Performance Scale (PPSv2), copyright Victoria Hospice Society

PPS Level	Ambulation	Activity & Evidence of Disease	Self-Care	Intake	Conscious Level
100%	Full	Normal activity & work No evidence of disease	Full	Normal	Full
90%	Full	Normal activity & work Some evidence of disease	Full	Normal	Full
80%	Full	Normal activity with effort Some evidence of disease	Full	Normal or reduced	Full
70%	Reduced	Unable normal job/work Significant disease	Full	Normal or reduced	Full
60%	Reduced	Unable hobby/house work Significant disease	Occasional assistance necessary	Normal or reduced	Full or confusion
50%	Mainly sit/lie	Unable to do any work Extensive disease	Considerable assistance required	Normal or reduced	Full or confusion
40%	Mainly in bed	Unable to do most activity Extensive disease	Mainly assistance	Normal or reduced	Full or drowsy +/- confusion
30%	Totally bed bound	Unable to do any activity Extensive disease	Total care	Normal or reduced	Full or drowsy +/- confusion
20%	Totally bed bound	Unable to do any activity Extensive disease	Total care	Minimal to sips	Full or drowsy +/- confusion
10%	Totally bed bound	Unable to do any activity Extensive disease	Total care	Mouth care only	Drowsy or coma +/- confusion
0%	Death	–	–	–	–

The ER staff conveyed the situation to hospice, and the hospice doctor determined it was fine to release Mom. We found a nurse who assisted us in the back-and-forth discussions, my sister-in-law made a few phone calls, and we finally got Mom admitted to the hospital, where she stayed for about a week. By the time we got her home, she had all the equipment she needed, including a wheelchair and a hospital bed.

She never really got out of the wheelchair for any length of time after she left the hospital until she passed away. It took a long time to get her any physical therapy at all. Hospice did not want to order it as it was not related to her Alzheimer's progression, and other doctors were averse to ordering it (or could not) because she was under hospice care. Her muscles would keep getting weaker the longer she stayed in the chair and received no physical therapy.

At this point, we started having the caregiver come to the house five or six days a week. I physically could not handle transferring Mom from bed to wheelchair to couch and back again, plus at least a few additional transfers during the day for toileting.

The hospice nurse visited with Mom weekly throughout the months that followed; the certified nursing assistant visited more often for bed and bath care; the doctor visited on critical occasions; the social worker and chaplain visited about once a month; and the music therapist came one or two times a month.

Excerpts from the notes from these visits show Mom's rapid decline from February 17 ("Pt remains weak and needs max assist for transfer and standing. Appetite is improving but has to be fed.") to March 16 ("Decline in appetite. Obvious weight loss with evidence of loosely fitting clothes and wasting muscle.") to April 11 ("While this nurse practitioner attempted to engage the patient in the conversation, the patient answered every question with a one or two word statement that was incorrect. She was able to briefly maintain eye contact.") to April 13 when the hospice doctor visited ("The patient has difficulty swallowing. The patient has tremors. She is sleeping more and more. The patient is weak and frail. It is unlikely that the patient will survive 6 months.").

On April 27, 2017, Mom and I were sitting on the couch. I was giving her some mashed sweet potatoes (she was only eating pureed food at this point, because the medical staff was concerned about aspiration), when she seemed to have what I thought was a seizure or stroke. Her left arm shot out and remained there very stiff for a bit. She began severely vomiting. One eye was locked in a gaze pointing outward. When I tried to straighten her a bit, she remained very stiff. I called 911 and the paramedics came again and took Mom to the hospital nearby that was equipped to treat seizures and strokes if that is what it turned out to be.

Mom was admitted to the initial hospital on April 27. They completed a computerized tomography and magnetic resonance imaging of Mom's brain, which were negative for any acute stroke. The hospital notes conveyed that the involuntary twitching Mom was experiencing was likely related to dementia with Parkinsonian features.

On April 28, Mom was transferred to a second hospital's hospice unit. On April 30, the notes from the hospital convey the following:

April 30, 2017
Over the past 12 hours patient has required two doses of Ativan for acute anxiety and tremulousness. Patient visibly distraught on exam today with tremulousness and poor appetite. Patient denied any acute pain. She was not oriented to place or time but was oriented to person. Goals of care remain comfort measures only. I have increased patient's Remeron to 30 mg. Will continue Ativan for breakthrough anxiety. I suspect patient will likely need bridge of anxiolytics until antidepressant therapy becomes effective. Daughter updated on condition and plan of care. Given decline in functional status the patient's overall prognosis remains grim and the patient is to remain here in the unit for symptom management, specifically her anxiety and agitation. Will consider discharge should patient's symptoms improve or stabilize.

On May 2, 2017 Mom was released from the hospital's hospice unit and transferred home. She continued to decline after this hospital stay. Eventually, on May 13, the Trustbridge team advised that Mom would be more comfortable staying in bed. They provided an air mattress that readjusts automatically and helps to prevent bedsores and they gave us an oxygen tank for when Mom needed it. Mom was only eating pureed food and very little overall.

Hospice was visiting regularly at home. The following notes were made by the hospice team in the month following Mom's discharge from the hospital.

June 2, 2017

This is a frail elderly female who is lying in bed with eyes closed. She is non-verbal and no interactions during this visit. She has to be fed. And takes more than 1 hour to eat a meal. Has significant dysphagia and takes a pureed diet. She has to be spoon fed. She sometimes pockets food and needs cueing to swallow. High risk for aspirations. Incontinent of bladder and bowel. Foley catheter draining. Rigidity to extremities. Chronic pain to shoulders. Requires total care. PPS 30%.

June 16, 2017

Pt lying in bed with eyes closed. Pt responded in weak tone yes/no. Pt is pale and weak, bed bound and requiring total ADL care. Appetite poor, occasional coughing during meals and intake has decreased. Pt has no pain. Foley cath insitu and drained 200ccs amber colored urine. Daughter requesting crisis care. Explained the criteria of which pt is not meeting. Daughter tearful. EOL care and expectation reviewed with daughter. Understands.

Seven days after the June 16 entry, Mom was admitted into hospice crisis care, which meant that hospice staff would now be at the home around-the-clock.

In the last several months of Mom's life, hospice care seemed like the right step. Prior to that time, another option for her care, palliative care, was not mentioned by anyone as something we might explore. It is important, however, that people impacted by Alzheimer's disease know about palliative care, and the difference between it and hospice.

The NIH National Institute on Aging summarizes the difference between palliative care and hospice care:[1] They note that palliative care, which can be helpful at any stage of illness and is best provided from the point of diagnosis, is a resource for anyone living with a serious illness, such as heart failure, cancer, dementia, Parkinson's disease, and many others. Palliative care can improve quality of life, help with symptoms, and help patients understand their choices for medical treatment. Palliative care recognizes that a serious illness affects more than just the body. It touches all areas of a person's life, as well as lives of that person's family members. Palliative care can address these effects of a person's illness: physical problems; emotional, social, and coping problems; practical problems; and spiritual issues. Palliative care can be provided along with curative treatment and does not depend on prognosis.

Like palliative care, hospice provides comprehensive comfort care as well as support for the family, but, in hospice, attempts to cure the person's illness are stopped. Hospice is provided for a person with a terminal illness whose doctor believes he or she has six months or less to live if the illness runs its natural course. Hospice is an approach to care that can take place at home or in a facility.

The American Board of Medical Specialties (ABMS) defines this subspecialty practice area as Hospice and Palliative Medicine (HPM). Since 2008, member boards of ABMS and AOA (American Osteopathic Association Bureau of Osteopathic Specialists) have certified 8,197 physicians in the specialty-level practice of hospice and palliative medicine. The vast majority of new HPM physicians (82.4%) are providing HPM patient care services, according to a January 2019 report.[2]

In an interview with National Public Radio (NPR) in 2013, Dr. Porter Storey, past executive vice president of the American Academy of Hospice and Palliative Medicine, said, "In Europe or Canada or Australia, hospice care and palliative care are the same thing. But in this country, the Medicare hospice benefit has defined hospice care as a wonderful set of services, but only for people in their last six months of life."[3]

Palliative Care

The World Health Organization (WHO) reports that each year an estimated 40 million people are in need of palliative care, 78% of them are people who live in low- and middle-income countries. Worldwide, only about 14% of people who need palliative care currently receive it.[4]

According to the 2019 report "America's Care of Serious Illness: A State by State Report Card on Access to Palliative Care in our Nation's Hospitals:"

> America's health care delivery system does not currently meet the needs of patients and families living with a serious illness. Our nation's focus on disease-specific treatments, rather than on the needs of the whole person and their family, has resulted in unnecessary suffering, fragmented, burdensome—often futile—and costly interventions, untreated pain and symptoms, lengthy and repeated hospitalizations and emergency department visits, overwhelmed family caregivers, and clinician burnout.[5]

The report continues to note that 94% of U.S. hospitals with more than 300 beds now have a palliative care team, compared to 62% of hospitals with 50 to 299 beds. There is also variability based upon region with East South Central (Alabama, Kentucky, Mississippi, and Tennessee) and West South Central (Arkansas, Louisiana, Oklahoma, and Texas) regions having the lowest levels of such service. New England (Connecticut, Maine, Massachusetts, New Hampshire, Rhode Island, and Vermont), Mid-Atlantic (New Jersey, New York, Pennsylvania), and East North Central (Illinois, Indiana, Michigan, Ohio, Wisconsin) regions have the highest levels of such service. The states with the lowest ratings for service of this kind are

Alabama, Mississippi, Oklahoma, New Mexico, and Wyoming. The states with 100% of large hospitals offering such care are New Hampshire, Rhode Island, Vermont, and Delaware.

Along with progress in the growth of the palliative care practice, there has been progress in the identification of quality standards for palliative care, and possible funding avenues through Medicare. In 2018, the fourth edition of the National Consensus Project (NCP) *Clinical Practice Guidelines for Quality Palliative Care* was published, updating existing guidelines and establishing new standards and expectations for all health care professionals caring for people living with a serious illness and their families.[6]

In the last three years, Medicare has made changes to allow specific payment for advance care planning and complex chronic care management. The Center for Medicare and Medicaid Innovation (CMMI) began testing new models that expand access to palliative care specialists, including the Oncology Care Model and the Medicare Care Choices Model. The Creating High-Quality Results and Outcomes Necessary to Improve Chronic (CHRONIC) Care Act, passed as part of the Bipartisan Budget Act of 2018, will allow Medicare Advantage (MA) plans to pay for social supports as well as in-home palliative care services for specific populations. Value-based insurance design may also provide a payment platform for nonhospital palliative care.

Get Palliative Care (www.getpalliativecare.org) provides a state-by-state list of palliative care providers, and a quiz to find out if it's a fit for a particular situation (https://getpalliativecare.org/rightforyou). Ask your doctor if you think palliative care may be an option for you or your loved one.

Hospice Care

The National Hospice and Palliative Care Organization (NHPCO) describes hospice care as follows:[7]

> Considered to be the model for quality, compassionate care at the end of life, hospice care involves a team-oriented

approach of expert medical care, pain management, and emotional and spiritual support tailored to the patient's needs and wishes. Support is provided to the patient's loved ones as well.

The National Hospice and Palliative Care Organization (NHPCO), the largest nonprofit membership organization representing hospice and palliative care programs and professionals in the United States, recently reported in the "NHPCO Facts and Figures: 2018 Edition" that over the course of 2017, there were 4,515 Medicare-certified hospices in operation. The greatest percentage of days of care while in hospice were spent at home (56%), with 42.7% of days spent in a nursing facility. Cancer represented the greatest percentage of diagnoses of those in hospice at 30.1%; dementia represented 15.6%. Dementia patients had the highest average of number of days spent in hospice at 110 days; cancer, by comparison, was 48 days.[8]

As noted previously, Medicare provides coverage for hospice care (see a summary of these benefits in its publication *Medicare Hospice Benefits*[9]). The Medicare Hospice Benefit affords patients four levels of care to meet their clinical needs: Routine Hospice Care, General Inpatient Care, Continuous Home Care, and Inpatient Respite Care. Payment for each covers all aspects of the patient's care related to the terminal illness, including all services delivered by the interdisciplinary team, medications, medical equipment, and supplies.

Routine Hospice Care (RHC) is the most common level of hospice care. With this type of care, an individual has elected to receive hospice care at their residence. General Inpatient Care (GIP) is provided for pain control or other acute symptom management that cannot feasibly be provided in any other setting. GIP begins when other efforts to manage symptoms are not sufficient. GIP can be provided in a Medicare-certified hospital, hospice inpatient facility, or nursing facility that has a registered nurse available 24 hours a day to provide direct patient care. Continuous Home Care (CHC) is care provided for between 8 and 24 hours a day to manage pain and other acute medical symptoms. CHC services must be predominately nursing care, supplemented with caregiver and hospice aide services, and are intended to maintain the terminally ill patient at home during a pain or symptom crisis. Inpatient Respite Care (IRC) is available to provide temporary relief to the patient's primary caregiver. Respite care can be provided in a hospital, hospice facility, or a long-term care facility that has sufficient 24-hour nursing personnel present. If the usual caregiver (like a family member) needs rest, the patient can get inpatient respite care in a Medicare-approved facility (like a hospice inpatient facility, hospital, or nursing home) for up to five days each time.

Medicare.gov also provides a "Hospice Compare" service that allows the user to search and find out information for a specific hospice organization or to compare a number of organizations in a certain area (via search by zip code, city, or state).[10] For example, a search for Florida yields 49 results, with their for-profit or nonprofit status, contact information, and date of certification. Comparisons of different organizations provide family caregivers' survey responses on family experience of care, patient preferences, and managing pain and treating symptoms.

What Next?

1. Determine if your health insurance covers palliative care and hospice care. Medicare covers hospice care; coverage for palliative care in the United States is not as certain.
2. If you think that palliative care or hospice care is needed, ask the primary doctor or specialist how to move forward. Remember, you know the situation better than anyone, so you may need to inform a doctor more fully as to why you think these services may be needed at the time.
3. Visit www.getpalliativecare.org for more information on palliative care in your area.
4. Visit Medicare.gov for the "Hospice Compare" service to research hospice services in your area.

5. Once receiving hospice services, understand that the hospice physician will be the primary point of contact for oversight of medical decisions. Be sure to talk with your general practitioner and/or specialist to understand what this means.

6. Have discussions as early in the disease process as possible regarding wishes in the final stages of life. Discuss things such as DNR (Do Not Resuscitate orders), life support, etc., to best understand what is desired. When admitted into hospice, one of the first things a person is asked about is whether there is a DNR. If not, one is provided for consideration and signature by the responsible party and the hospice doctor. Hospice will advise to keep the DNR visible in your home, so if emergency medical assistance is ever needed, the team is aware of the DNR.

7. Understand that a person in the final stages of illness may experience pain and cannot move or be moved a great deal. If admitted into hospice, the hospice team will monitor pain, ensure medication is provided as needed, and secure any other equipment that might help. For example, a hospital bed is often needed. It is important to know that there are beds available that have the motion needed to reduce pressure points and help in preventing bed sores. And, while it is not something most people would naturally think of, anyone who loves someone in this situation should understand that once he or she is in a hospital bed and in pain, you will not be able to do something as simple and loving as lay next to your loved one. Side-by-side hospital beds or a bed at the same elevation as the hospital bed can be a good option to keep your loved one comfortable and maintain your ability to comfort them.

CHAPTER 9

DEATH

Trust in the Lord with all thine heart;
and lean not unto thine own understanding.
In all thy ways acknowledge Him and
He shall direct thy paths.
—*Proverbs 3:5–6 (KJV)*

Early in Mom's disease, she bought a plaque with Proverbs 3:5–6 on it. "Mom, where should we hang this?" I asked her one day. "Next to my bed where I can see it."

A few months later, after Mom's official diagnosis, we would look at the plaque and read it together most nights when she went to bed. When she could no longer read herself, I read it for her. Although she was always quiet about it, Mom had her faith to sustain and support her through every difficult step of this disease. Out of us reading this plaque together on so many occasions throughout the disease, when Mom was having a very hard time, I would have nothing left to say but "Give it to God." She would take a deep breath, and then did.

On June 23, 2017, when the nurse came for her visit, we decided it was time for Mom to have round-the-clock hospice crisis care in the home. Because the nurse was not there with Mom every day and unable to see how little she ate or drank, or how much pain she seemed to be in at times, I had to convince the nurse it was time. "If this isn't the time for critical care, then tell me, when is?" I asked.

Mom was in bed around the clock, she was no longer opening her eyes and, to get her to eat, her caregiver sat patiently next to her bed for hours on end, trying to just get her to have one more spoonful of anything—even just ice cream, which was always Mom's favorite. She also would screech whenever her caregiver tried to move her even an inch to give her a very gentle bed bath.

The following notes were made to her file on the day Mom entered crisis care and three days later when the doctor visited:

June 23, 2017

Pt has reduced alertness, kept eyes closed. 1–2 words but mainly sleeping with mouth open. Pt grimacing and groaning in pain. Pt has increased swallowing problems, coughing on food and drink. Upper lungs have scattered rhonchi. Some difficulty breathing. Spoke to dr who started pt on crisis care for pain and ineffective breathing.

June 26, 2017

The patient is lying down on the hospital bed. She is using oxygen with a nasal cannula. The patient is semicomatose. She is not responsive. The history is obtained from the patient's daughter and the patient's crisis care nurse. The patient was started on crisis care 3 days ago by this physician because of ineffective breathing. The breathing difficulties escalated over the past several days. Morphine was changed to around the clock from p.r.n. dosing … She is poorly responsive. The crisis care nurse informs me that earlier today the patient did open one eye. She stared blankly into space. She then closed her eyes. The patient at times has pain. This occurs mostly when care is provided to her. She will then frown and grimace …

Assessment: The patient is imminent. Her PPS is 10.

PLAN: Morphine will be continued around the clock and as needed at a dose of 4 mg. Atropine and the Ativan will be given as needed to treat their respective symptoms. The Transderm scopolamine patch will be continued to treat the congestion. Advanced directives and do not resuscitate were discussed with the family and crisis care nurse. Prognosis is poor. I informed the family and crisis care nurse that the patient is semicomatose. I informed the family that the patient can still hear us and will be able to do so until the very end ... I explained to the family the agitation is secondary to terminal agitation which is commonly seen at the end of life in terminally ill patients. The patient is terminal as she has a history of senile degeneration of the brain. Her course was complicated by semicoma, dyspnea, congestion, pain, agitation.

Mom passed away on June 29, 2017, at 9:35 p.m. in her bed at home.

It was six days after she was admitted to crisis care.

Her breaths just came further and further apart until she did not take another breath.

My sister-in-law was holding one of Mom's hands. I was holding the other.

The moment she passed, she felt cold.

It felt like she was immediately no longer there—in her body.

It was the worst moment of my life.

I wailed as I have never done.

And never will again.

When a person is diagnosed with Alzheimer's disease, they and their loved ones usually understand that the disease is fatal. They generally know the person with Alzheimer's can live for years after the diagnosis, but that his or her physical and mental state will continue to decline. Often, though, people do not know about all the ways that Alzheimer's will affect the physical body in the later stages of the disease. They also may expect that, with years between diagnosis and death, they might be better prepared for death. I, for one, was not prepared. Perhaps knowing more would have helped—even just a bit.

Deaths due to dementia worldwide have more than doubled between 2000 and 2016, making it the fifth leading global cause of death in 2016, compared to fourteenth in 2000. Alzheimer's disease and other dementias are among the top ten causes of death in upper-middle and high-income countries; it is not among the top ten in low-income and lower-middle income countries.[1]

The countries with the highest death rates from Alzheimer's and dementias, in order from the highest, are Finland, Kuwait, Turkey, Saudi Arabia, United Kingdom, Tunisia, Libya, United States, Syria, and Lebanon. The countries with the lowest death rates from Alzheimer's and dementias, in order from the lowest, are Singapore, Kyrgyzstan, Philippines, Macedonia, Uzbekistan, Mauritius, Columbia, Ukraine, Saint Lucia, and Venezuela.[2]

Alzheimer's disease and other dementias remained the leading cause of death in England and Wales in 2017 (the third consecutive year), accounting for 12.7% of all deaths registered.[3] In the United States, Alzheimer's disease is officially listed as the sixth-leading cause of death. It is the fifth-leading cause of death for those ages 75 to 84, and the third-leading cause of death for those 85 and older.[4]

Alzheimer's, as a cause of death in the United States, increased 55% from 1999 to 2014. The number of Alzheimer's deaths at home increased from 14% to 25%, while deaths in institutional settings decreased from 1999 to 2014.[5]

The increase of Alzheimer's deaths and the proportion of those deaths occurring at home has increased the burden on caregivers. With more deaths occurring at home, it can help to know what to expect in advance. No two deaths will ever be the same, but having some understanding of what is common (or not) may be helpful. The following are the signs that often precede death.[6]

One to three months before death, a person is likely to sleep or doze more, eat and drink less, withdraw from people and stop doing things they used to enjoy, and talk less.

One to two weeks before death, the person may feel tired and drained all the time, so much that they don't leave their bed. He or she could have different sleep-wake patterns; little appetite and thirst; fewer and smaller bowel movements and less urinating; more pain; changes in blood pressure, breathing, and heart rate; body temperature ups and downs that may leave their skin cool, warm, moist, or pale; congested breathing from the buildup in the back of the throat; confusion or seeming to be in a daze; and hallucinations and visions, especially of long-gone loved ones.

When death is within days or hours, a person may not want food or drink; stop urinating and having bowel movements; grimace, groan, or scowl from pain; have his or her eyes tear or glaze over; have an irregular or hard to find pulse and heartbeat; have a drop in body temperature; have skin on their knees, feet, and hands turn a mottled bluish-purple (often in the last 24 hours); and drift in and out of consciousness, if they are not already unconscious.

The final stages of dying will likely involve changes in breathing. One such change is called Cheyne-Stokes breathing, a cycle of 30 seconds to two minutes when breathing deepens and speeds up, then gets shallower and shallower until it stops. Then, there is a pause, which can last long enough that it seems the person has stopped breathing altogether—and then the cycle continues.

Some people may make a different type of sound as they breathe, caused by a buildup of saliva or secretions at the back of the throat. This happens because the dying person is not clearing their throat or swallowing. It can also sound like there is congestion in the dying person's lungs.

While the dying person may be unresponsive, there is growing evidence that even in this unconscious state, people are aware of what is going on around them and can hear conversations and words spoken to them, although it may feel to them like they are in a dream state.

After Death

If a person is dying at home and does not want CPR, calling 911 is not necessary. In fact, a call to 911 could cause confusion. Many places require emergency medical technicians (EMTs) who respond to 911 calls to perform CPR if someone's heart has stopped. Consider having a nonhospital DNR (Do Not Resuscitate order) if the person is dying at home. A hospice team will ensure this happens or, in absence of hospice care, ask the primary physician to assist with it. Also, determine in advance who to call after the death by asking the doctor or the hospice care team.

The National Health Institute (NHI) National Institute on Aging (NIA) also provides advice.[7] For example, they advise that nothing has to be done immediately after a person's death. Take the time you need. Some people want to stay in the room with the body; others prefer to leave. You might want to have someone make sure the body is lying flat before the joints become stiff and cannot be moved. This rigor mortis begins sometime during the first hours after death. After the death, how long you can stay with the body may depend on where the death happens. If it happens at home, there is no need to move the body right away. This is the time for any special religious, ethnic, or cultural customs that are performed soon after death.

In addition, those providing care should know that, as soon as possible, the death must be officially pronounced by someone in authority, like a doctor in a hospital or nursing facility or a hospice nurse. This person also fills out the forms certifying the cause, time, and place of death. These steps will make it possible for an official death certificate to be prepared. If hospice is helping, a plan for what happens after death is already in place. If death happens at home without hospice, try to talk with the doctor, local medical examiner (coroner), your local health department, or a funeral home representative in advance about how to proceed.

Arrangements should be made to pick up the body as soon as the family is ready and according to local laws. Usually, this is done by a funeral home.

The hospital or nursing facility, if that is where the death took place, may call the funeral home for you. If at home, contact the funeral home directly or ask a friend or family member to do it. The doctor may ask if you want an autopsy. This is a medical procedure conducted by a specially trained physician to learn more about what caused the death. For example, if the person who died was believed to have Alzheimer's disease, a brain autopsy will allow for a definitive diagnosis. If your religion or culture objects to autopsies, talk to the doctor. Some people planning a funeral with a viewing worry about having an autopsy, but the physical signs of an autopsy are usually hidden by clothing.

Organ Donation Considerations

In addition to any consideration of autopsy, you or your loved one may have indicated a desire for organ donation. Alzheimer's disease does not necessarily exclude someone from organ donation. Since patients with Alzheimer's are usually older, individual assessment is necessary. Heart and lung recovery from older-age donors is rare, for example. Overall, medical condition at time of death determines what organs and tissues can be donated.

It is important to know that if the person has requested a DNR but wants to donate organs, he or she may have to indicate that the desire to donate supersedes the DNR. That is because it might be necessary to use machines to keep the heart beating until the medical staff is ready to remove the donated organs. Learn more about potential organ, eye, and tissue donation at www.donatelife.net.

Brain donation is different from other organ donation. As an organ donor, you agree to give your organs to other people to help keep them alive. As a brain donor, your brain will be used for research purposes only. Scientists use brain tissue donated after death to better understand the causes of and treatment options for Alzheimer's disease and related dementias.

The National Institute on Aging (NIA) funds Alzheimer's Disease Research Centers (ADRCs) at major medical institutions across the

United States. The NIA website provides a link to locate ADRCs near you (https://www.nia.nih.gov/health/alzheimers-disease-research-centers).[8] These ADRCs work with individuals who want to make brain donations. Any person wanting to make a brain donation needs to begin the process early, as advance preparation is required. In addition, sometimes these centers only accept donations from those who have participated in a research study at their center.

The NIA outlines the steps that are needed for brain donation:[9]

Step 1: Enroll in the brain donation program with an Alzheimer's Disease Research Center (ADRC).

Step 2: Sign a consent form with the ADRC.

Step 3: Designate a family member or other representative to contact the ADRC at the time of death. It is important that the center is contacted immediately, ideally within two hours of death.

Step 4: The ADRC will assist your loved ones in making arrangements for transportation to and from the donation site.

Step 5: The brain removal is performed.

Step 6: The brain autopsy is performed. Brain tissue is stored in a carefully controlled Brain Bank.

Step 7: Your family or other designated recipient is notified with the results of the brain autopsy. This may take up to six months.

Step 8: Brain tissue is available to qualified scientists across the country for critical research.

The NIA currently lists 32 Alzheimer's Disease Centers (ADCs) across the country that conduct Alzheimer's research (it is important to visit the NIA website for an updated lists of ADCs). As an example, in Florida, there are two ADCs listed: Mayo Clinic Memory Disorder Clinic in Jacksonville (www.mayo.edu/research/centers-programs/alzheimers-disease-research-center; 904-953-6523) and the University of Florida Alzheimer's Disease Center in Gainesville (http://1floridaadrc.org; 352-273-7436).

In addition to the ADCs, the National Institutes of Health (NIH) NeuroBioBank program includes six banks that accept donations from individuals with neurological disorders resulting in dementia, including, but not limited to, vascular, frontotemporal, and Lewy body dementia (LBD). Individuals diagnosed with Alzheimer's disease are referred to the Alzheimer's Disease Centers program, as space at the brain banks is limited. The six brain banks currently listed on the NIH website include:[10]

- University of Maryland Brain and Tissue Bank (800.847.1539; btbumab@umaryland.edu; accepts donations from all states except Hawaii; does not accept Alzheimer's donations).
- Brain Endowment Bank, University of Miami (800.862.7246; accepts donations from most states; does not accept Alzheimer's donations).
- The Human Brain and Spinal Fluid Resource Center (310.268.3536; brainbnk@ucla.edu; accepts donations from most states; does not accept Alzheimer's donations).
- Harvard Brain Tissue Resource Center (800.272.4622; accepts donations from all states except Alaska, Mississippi, and Oklahoma; does not accept Alzheimer's donations).
- Mount Sinai NIH Brain and Tissue Repository (718.584.9000 ext.6083; NBTR@mssm.edu, accepts donations only from New Jersey, New York, and Pennsylvania; unknown whether Alzheimer's donations are accepted).
- Brain Tissue Donation Program at the University of Pittsburgh (412.624.7802; johnstoncs@upmc.edu; unknown whether Alzheimer's donations are accepted).

Other facilities that accept brain donations from individuals with Alzheimer's disease or other dementias include:

- The Veterans Affairs (VA) Biorepository Brain Bank (866.460.1158; accepts donations from veterans across the United States, including Alzheimer's donations).
- National Disease Research Interchange (800.222.6374; accepts donations from across the United States, including Alzheimer's donations).
- Brown Brain Tissue Resource Center (401.444.5155; accepts donations from those who were patients of Brown University physicians).
- Oregon Brain Bank (503.494.0100; woltjerr@ohsu.edu; accepts donations from Oregon residents; may accept Alzheimer's donations depending on current needs).
- Virginia Commonwealth University Brain Tissue Resource Facility (804.828.9664; pdcbtrf@vcuhealth.org; accepts whole-body donations that can be received within 18 hours of death).

The National Cell Repository for Alzheimer's Disease (NCRAD https:// ncrad.iu.edu) also provides opportunities for potential donation. The goal of the NCRAD is to help researchers find genes that increase the risk for Alzheimer's disease and other dementias. The NCRAD provides researchers with biological samples (such as DNA, plasma, serum, RNA, cerebrospinal fluid, cell lines, and brain tissue) for study. The NCRAD enrolls families into its programs. Its programs include, among other efforts, a bank for brain donations and clinical trials in which family members may be eligible to participate. To make a brain donation, an individual must have two or more living blood relatives with symptoms of Alzheimer's or another dementia. These symptomatic relatives must be willing to donate a biological sample (blood or saliva) before death and provide the NCRAD with their medical records. If the individual inquiring about brain donation has dementia, only one blood relative is needed. The NCRAD accepts donations from all states.

As discussed, if donation (brain or otherwise) is a desired direction, it is important to research and plan for this well in advance. The process

typically requires several steps and, in some cases, requires advance participation in a research effort in order to donate.

What Next?

1. If the dying person will be at home for the days preceding death and
    at the time of death, make sure that the environment is as they would
    want. If they love music, have it playing as often as possible. If they
    love having family and friends around, have them there when possible.
    Touch them and hold their hands. Doctors will tell you that hearing is
    the last sense to go, so talk to them. Read to them.
2. If the dying person will be at home at the time of death, make sure you
    know what steps to take, or have someone else prepared to take them. If
    the person will be in a facility where medical care is available, there will
    be people to advise you.
3. If the dying person will be at home at the time of death, and it was
    decided that they did not want any life-saving measures, it is important
    that you have a DNR at the home. If the person will be in another
    facility, make sure that facility has a copy of the DNR.
4. If the person indicated that they desired to be an organ donor or,
    specifically, a brain donor, in the months prior to death, ensure that all
    arrangements that are needed have been made. At the time of death,
    you will need to take the steps agreed to in advance, depending on the
    specifics of the donation.
5. Have all funeral arrangements made in advance. When you do, all
    you will need to do is call the funeral home and they will take care of
    everything for you.

CHAPTER 10

GRIEF

Grief is the price we pay for love.
—*Queen Elizabeth II*

Having the people arrive to the house after Mom's passing to take her to a nearby funeral home was awful and surreal. My husband kept trying to pull me away from Mom and from watching as they took Mom out. As they could not get a cot around the corner into the bedroom, I watched as they had to push Mom out on a dolly. She was wrapped in a white sheet, tucked very tightly around her body and face. The two men who came pushed the dolly out the door and moved Mom into the plain white van they came in. My brother, sister-in-law, niece, husband, and I followed them out the door. It was all I could do to not climb in that van with her. I did not want her in that van with two strangers driving. I did not want her to be put into the bottom of a plane for the travel back to Pennsylvania for the funeral.

All we could do was watch as the van pulled away.

Mom's funeral service happened very quickly, mostly because everything had been prepared in advance. Mom passed on a Thursday night, June 29, 2017.

The visitation at the funeral home was on Sunday. The funeral was on Monday, July 3, 2017.

Among the people who spoke to celebrate Mom at her funeral was her granddaughter, my brother's youngest daughter. Here is what she said:

> Many people never have the privilege to meet someone with genuine care and love for everyone. I was fortunate enough to meet someone like that. Not only was she my grandma, but she was also my best friend. If you knew my grandma and I, you knew the inseparable bond her and I shared. From long talks on the phone at night after spending the whole day with her, to getting Carvel ice cream after she picked me up from school, I knew our love for each other was everlasting. Wherever you went, nothing but smiles followed. Your smile was the most amazing sight I have ever seen. It was the only thing that could comfort me on my toughest days. You were the person who opened my eyes to all the positivity that's out there because you always saw the good in everybody. You were the type of lady to literally give your clothes off your back. I remember always telling you that I loved your shirt and you would always say, "Do you want it?" That's just the kind of heart and love she had for others. I know that if anyone belonged in heaven, she surely did. As I continue life in Orlando, I promise that I will make you proud and will not let you down. I want you to know that every achievement and accomplishment I make, I will look up at you and say, "I did it, Grandma," just as if you were still here with me. You may not be here physically but you are in my heart and your legacy will carry on through me. And I will always continue to have those long talks with you. You were the strongest person I have ever met. Not once did I ever see you close to giving up. You fought harder than I thought possible, but at 9:35 p.m. Thursday night, God took

you away from us. You lost the battle against Alzheimer's.
You're no longer suffering and no longer in pain. Your spirit is
set free and you're in a better place. I love you Grandma—my
guardian angel.

After the funeral, I spent more than two years in my own private crisis.

I cried uncontrollably almost every day for the first year. When the tears and sobs came for so long and so consistently, pretty soon, gasping for breath was a reflex—trying to exhale for your life and for missing your loved one so much.

There were many, many days that I did not want to get out of bed, and I did not. I had stopped working to care for my mother, and I could not find the consistent strength and motivation to begin working again. I was trying, but the sadness kept pulling me away from the productive life I had before. I just wanted to sleep.

After the first three months or so, my husband would say that it was time to move on—that people lose someone they love all of the time, and they work through it. I needed to work through it too.

I tried to explain that this did not feel like "normal" grief (if there is such a thing). I lost my mother and my best friend, but having cared for her for so long, I almost felt as if I had lost a child, too. And I had watched Mom die, as well as been there through the very awful process that preceded it. Memories of this time were the memories that were haunting me the most.

Hospice offered grief support to the family of those who passed while in their care, and I visited with a grief counselor twice. I remember one conversation in particular.

"Do you feel like a victim—helpless?" she asked me.

"No, I don't feel helpless. I feel lost," I said.

She talked to me about how I had given up my work when I took care of Mom—given up everything that characterized who I was before. She talked about losing my own identity through this process to replace it with the identity of being Mom's caregiver. Now that Mom was gone, I did not have either identity any longer.

I only saw this counselor twice. At the time, I did not have the motivation to visit again, I suppose. But I continued to feel lost for two years after Mom's death. Some days, I felt so bad that I did not want to live.

Mostly when I felt this way, I was remembering the very difficult and heart-breaking experiences I had with Mom during her illness. I would relive the experience in my mind, remember how she looked at me, what she said, and what I did or did not do. Sometimes, I was thinking how much I missed my mother or about my purpose in life. Many years before, when I was a young adult, when I thought about purpose, I did not think about anything related to a career, even though I was extremely dedicated to mine. For whatever reason, I always thought first that my purpose was to be a good daughter. I think I must have known somewhere in my soul that I would be called on to realize that purpose in a fundamental, life-changing way.

Now I had cared for my mother in that way. I did not know what my purpose would or could be moving forward, or if I even had a purpose anymore.

Once, a month after Mom's passing, I met her caregiver for lunch. We cried together and remembered Mom together. She shared with me that she saw Mom in a dream shortly after Mom's death, and Mom was smiling and laughing and so happy. I told her about how much I was struggling, how the bad memories kept coming back, how I kept wondering if I had made mistakes in caring for Mom. Should I have done this or that differently?

She said, "Give it to God." She was telling me the same thing she had heard me say to my mother on more days than not. Mom's caregiver was caring for me. It was a gift. I was not as good at accepting it as was Mom.

Throughout the coming years, I continued to have horrible dreams. The place was always different and the people in the dream varied, but I was always with Mom. Mom wandered away and I lost her. In my dream, I kept yelling, "Mom! Mom! Mom!" I could never find her. She disappeared or, as I watched, disintegrated into nothing.

Today, as I'm finishing this book that I've worked on for over two years, I still miss my mother so much, but my knees buckle less and the days of uncontrolled sobbing are mostly gone. I can now think about how thankful I am to have had the mother I had and to have loved her so much. I can think of the good memories and smile now.

A cousin of my husband, whom I love, and who lost both her mom and dad, sent me a card after Mom's death that said on the front "God's gift of time." It talked about the time we need to heal. She already knew this. I was still learning.

I think time is the only way to heal. I also know that there is not a certain amount of time that every person needs to heal. Each person and experience are unique. Each person needs to take whatever time it takes to heal and to come back to life.

Elisabeth Kübler-Ross is very well-known for her stages of dying. David Kessler, who coauthored two books with her, also worked with her to adapt these stages for those in grief. Together they wrote the book titled, *On Grief and Grieving: Finding the Meaning of Grief Through the Five Stages of Loss.*[1]

In brief, the authors describe the five stages of grief as follows:

- **Denial**—This does not mean that you are denying the death of a loved one, but rather reflects the difficulty in knowing he or she will never physically be with you again. Believing that at this stage is too much.
- **Anger**—This is about being angry that you have to keep living in a world where your loved one is no longer present. The anger can be directed at anyone or everyone. Underneath it is the pain of loss or guilt (anger turned inward on yourself).
- **Bargaining**—After death, bargaining often moves from the past to the future. For example, we may bargain to see our loved ones again in heaven or in a dream.
- **Depression**—After bargaining, our attention turns to the present, and grief overtakes us at a deeper level—deeper than we ever imagined.

- **Acceptance**—This stage is about accepting the reality that our loved one is physically gone and recognizing that this new reality is the permanent reality.

Kübler-Ross and Kessler are careful to say that the stages of grief are responses to loss that many people have, but there is not a typical response to loss as there is no typical loss. The five stages—denial, anger, bargaining, depression, and acceptance—are a part of the framework that can help people make sense of what they are going through.

Not everyone goes through all the stages or goes through them in a prescribed order. Nor do the stages only happen after death. The authors explain that in long-term diseases like Alzheimer's disease, the loss of a loved one can be so gradual that there is time to experience all five stages even prior to death. Anticipatory grief occurs when a loved one has a terminal illness. Anticipatory grief feels like the "beginning of the end." Anticipatory grief is generally more silent than grief after a loss. People are often not as verbal. It is a grief people keep to themselves. Anticipatory grief stands alone from the grief after a loss. Even if a person goes through any or all of the five stages ahead of the death, they will still go through them again after the loss. "Anticipatory grief is just a prelude to the painful process we face, a double grief that will ultimately bring healing," say Kübler-Ross and Kessler.

The Center for Complicated Grief, part of the Columbia School of Social Work, specializes in a different type of grief, called complicated grief. They define complicated grief as "a persistent form of intense grief in which maladaptive thoughts and dysfunctional behaviors are present along with continued yearning, longing and sadness and/or preoccupation with thoughts and memories of the person who died. Grief continues to dominate life and the future seems bleak and empty. Irrational thoughts that the deceased person might reappear are common and the bereaved person feels lost and alone."[2]

The Mayo Clinic notes that while normal grief symptoms gradually start to fade over time, those of complicated grief linger or get worse.

Complicated grief is like being in an ongoing, heightened state of mourning that keeps you from healing. The risk of developing complicated grief, which occurs more often in females and with older age, may increase when the following factors are present:[3]

- an unexpected or violent death, such as death from a car accident or the murder or suicide of a loved one
- death of a child
- close or dependent relationship to the deceased person
- social isolation or loss of a support system or friendships
- past history of depression, separation anxiety, or post-traumatic stress disorder (PTSD)
- traumatic childhood experiences, such as abuse or neglect
- other major life stressors, such as major financial hardships

If the following symptoms are still present six months to a year after the death of a loved one, that can indicate grief has shifted into complicated grief:

- intense sorrow, pain, and rumination over the loss of your loved one
- focus on little else but your loved one's death
- extreme focus on reminders of the loved one or excessive avoidance of reminders
- intense and persistent longing or pining for the deceased
- problems accepting the death
- numbness or detachment
- bitterness about your loss
- feeling that life holds no meaning or purpose
- lack of trust in others
- inability to enjoy life or think back on positive experiences with your loved one
- having trouble carrying out normal routines

- isolation from others and withdrawing from social activities
- experiencing depression, deep sadness, guilt, or self-blame
- believing that you did something wrong or could have prevented the death
- feeling life isn't worth living without your loved one
- wishing you had died along with your loved one

The Mayo Clinic advises to contact a doctor or a mental health professional if this intense grief and symptoms are still present a year after the passing of a loved one.

The death of a loved one and the grief that follows it will represent a time in life unlike any other. There is so much sadness and darkness in that time, but there can also be tremendous renewal and light. Mother Teresa once said, "If only we could make people understand that we come from God and that we have to go back to Him! Death is the most decisive moment in human life. It is like our coronation: to die in peace with God."

At the end of the book, *On Grief and Grieving*, Kessler wrote:[4]

> Those whom we have loved and who loved us in return will always live on in our hearts and minds. As you continue on your journey, know that you are richer and stronger, and that you know yourself better now. You are transformed and evolved. You have loved, lost, and survived. You can find gratitude for the time you and your loved one shared together, as short as that seems to have been. Time helps as you continue healing and live on. Yours is the grace of life, death, and love.

What Next?

1. If you worked with a hospice organization, find out more about its grief counseling services and take advantage of them if you think it

could be helpful. Even if you are skeptical, give the service a try. These services are provided in the year after your loved one's death as part of the hospice program, and, therefore, are funded by Medicare.

2. Meeting with a counselor or therapist on an ongoing basis even after hospice-related services are not available, is important to consider.

3. Have someone whom you can talk to about your grief, whether a professional or a friend or relative, you will need the support and a listening ear.

4. Read books on grieving. I had studied the work of Kubler-Ross before my mother's death, but in reading her books again, I had a new, different, and very personal perspective regarding her learning and advice. I was amazed at how well her research mirrored my own grief process.

5. If religion is important to you, but you had gotten away from it because of care demands, consider if it is time to get involved again. Your religious leader may be another important confidante and advisor for you during this process.

6. Recognize that everyone grieves differently. Trust your own instincts and judgment about what will help you personally. Do not impose your own ideas on others about how one needs to grieve.

AFTERWORD

My mother, Sally Ann Sarber Baumgardner, was born on June 21, 1939. She was the fourth of James and Dorothy's five children.

They lived in a small white house in the tiny town an hour outside of Pittsburgh, Pennsylvania. The house had a front porch where Dorothy would often sit with her children, and then her children and grandchildren many years later. There was a small room in the front with an upright piano and a couch where Dorothy sat and knitted on many evenings. Off the kitchen, down the basement steps and out the back door, there was a long sloping yard. James's business was raising and selling chickens, so there were chicken coops stacked one on top of the other running almost the length of one side of the yard.

Mom's father died in 1951 at 41 years old with non-Hodgkin's lymphoma. She was 11. It is difficult to imagine the impact of the loss of her father on her at that age.

When James died, Dorothy was left with five children to raise. She had little time to grieve or relax and little money to spend for anything beyond the basic needs of her family. She worked hard, long hours in a drugstore for many years. She was an independent woman ahead of her time. Thin and striking, she had light blue eyes that always had a glint to them. She was strong. She was firm. She had a quick wit and a sometimes sharp tongue. She was not one to mince words. She went to church every Sunday and taught her children to be thoughtful and considerate—to always say please and thank you.

When my grandmother reached her seventies, even her strength was no match for the Alzheimer's disease that attacked her and led to her death in 1991 at the age of 76. As a young adult, I watched from afar as my step-grandfather, who married my grandmother in 1971, cared for my grandmother. He had no help at the time. Toward the end, he bathed her, washed her hair, cooked and fed her all of her meals, carried her up the stairs, dressed her, and took her out to visit with family and friends for as long as it was possible.

My mother's oldest brother died with Alzheimer's in 2006 at the age of 75. Her second brother died with Alzheimer's in 2012—one year before Mom was diagnosed. My mother's older sister died in her sleep at an earlier age (prior to the age when Alzheimer's typically appears). Her younger sister, who lives in a group home for developmentally disabled adults, just turned 69 this year.

A mother and three of her five children had all succumbed to the same terrible disease: Alzheimer's.

What should the children of these children expect?

What options do my brother, my sister, and I have to ensure we do not face the same future? What decisions can my seven cousins who had their fathers die with Alzheimer's make to help them prevent this disease?

My hope is that this book can inform this family of cousins, and many more outside of our family, about some of the steps we can take to help prevent the disease or to be better positioned to deal with it, should we ever have to come face-to-face with this monster.

Until there is a cure—there is something we can do.

NOTES

Chapter 1: Pre-diagnosis

1. Alzheimer's Association, "2012 Alzheimer's disease facts and figures," *Alzheimer's & Dementia*, 8 (2012): 131–168, https://doi.org/10.1016/j.jalz.2012.02.001.
2. Alzheimer's Disease International, *World Alzheimer's Report 2013—Journey of Caring: An Analysis of Long-term Care for Dementia*, https://www.alz.co.uk/research/WorldAlzheimerReport2013Executive Summary.pdf.
3. Alzheimer's Association, *2019 Alzheimer's Disease Facts and Figures*, https://www.alz.org/media/Documents/alzheimers-facts-and-figures-2019-r.pdf.
4. Liesi E. Hebert, Jennifer Weuve, Paul A. Scherr, and Denis A. Evans, "Alzheimer disease in the United States (2010–2050) estimated using the 2010 census," *Neurology* 80, no. 19 (2013): 1778–83, https://n.neurology.org/content/80/19/1778.
5. Alzheimer's Disease International, *World Alzheimer's Report 2018—The State of the Art of Dementia Research: New Frontiers*, https://www.alz.co.uk/research/WorldAlzheimerReport2018.pdf.
6. "What is Alzheimer's Disease?" National Institute on Aging, https://www.nia.nih.gov/health/what-alzheimers-disease.

7. See note 3 above.

8. See note 3 above.

9. Alzheimer's Disease International, *World Alzheimer's Report 2015—The Global Impact of Dementia: An Analysis of Prevalence, Incidence, Cost and Trends*, https://www.alz.co.uk/research/WorldAlzheimerReport2015.pdf.

10. Gus Bilirakis, "Congress should act on bipartisan legislation to address the devastating impact of Alzheimer's disease," *The Hill*, September 21, 2018, https://thehill.com/blogs/congress-blog/healthcare/407724-congress-should-act-on-bipartisan-legislation-to-address-the.

11. See note 3 above.

12. Gill Livingston, Andrew Sommerlad, Vasiliki Orgeta, Sergi G. Costafreda, Jonathan Huntley, David Ames, Clive Ballard, Sube Banerjee, Alistair Burns, Jiska Cohen-Mansfield, Claudia Cooper, Nick Fox, Laura N Gitlin, Robert Howard, Helen C. Kales, Eric B. Larson, Karen Ritchie, Kenneth Rockwood, Elizabeth L. Sampson, Quincy Samus, Lon S. Schneider, Geir Selbæk, Linda Teri, and Naaheed Mukadam, "Dementia prevention, intervention, and care," *The Lancet* 390, no. 10133 (2017): 2673–2734, doi: 10.1016/S0140-6736(17)31363-6.

13. David Watson, Psy.D., personal communication, February 21, 2020.

Chapter 2: Diagnostic Assessment

1. Clifford R. Jack, Jr., David A. Bennett, Kaj Blennow, Maria C. Carrillo, Billy Dunn, Samantha Budd Haeberlein, David M. Holtzman, William Jagust, Frank Jessen, Jason Karlawish, Enchi Liu, Jose Luis Molinuevo, Thomas Montine, Creighton Phelps, Katherine P. Rankin, Christopher C. Rowe, Philip Scheltens, Eric Siemers, Heather M. Snyder, and Reisa Sperling, "NIA-AA Research Framework: Toward a biological definition of Alzheimer's disease," *Alzheimer's & Dementia* 14 (4) (2018):

535–562, https://www.sciencedirect.com/science/article/pii/
S1552526018300724?via%3Dihub.

2. Dale E. Bredesen, MD, *The End of Alzheimer's: The First Program to Prevent and Reverse Cognitive Decline* (New York: Avery, 2017).

Chapter 3: Diagnostic Results

1. Alzheimer's Association: Alzheimer's Impact Movement, *Policy Brief: Early Detection and Diagnosis of Alzheimer's Dementia*, August 2017, https://alzimpact.org/img/Policy_Brief_Early_Detection_and_Diagnosis_Brief_AIM.pdf.

2. The Gerontological Society of America, *The Gerontological Society of America Workgroup on Cognitive Impairment Detection and Earlier Diagnosis: Report and Recommendations*, 2015, https://www.geron.org/images/gsa/documents/gsaciworkgroup2015report.pdf.

3. Alzheimer's Disease International (ADI), "Dementia Statistics," https://www.alz.co.uk/research/statistics.

4. Alzheimer's Association, "New Research Suggests Men Receive Misdiagnosis More Often Than Women," news release, July 26, 2016, https://www.alz.org/aaic/_downloads/Tues245ET-Clarifying-Misdiagnosis.pdf

5. Marwan N. Sabbagh, Lih-Fen Lue, Daniel Fayard, and Jiong Shi, "Increasing Precision of Clinical Diagnosis of Alzheimer's Disease Using a Combined Algorithm Incorporating Clinical and Novel Biomarker Data," *Neurology and Therapy* 6, no.1 (2017): 83–95, https://doi.org/10.1007/s40120-017-0069-5.

6. National Institute on Aging (NIA), "Symptoms and Diagnosis of Alzheimer's Disease: What are the Signs of Alzheimer's Disease?" https://www.nia.nih.gov/health/what-are-signs-alzheimers-disease.

7. Fisher Center for Alzheimer's Research Foundation, "Clinical Stages of Alzheimer's," https://www.alzinfo.org/understand-alzheimers/clinical-stages-of-alzheimers/.

Chapter 4: My Best Friend, Empathy, and Love

1. Virginia Bell and David Troxel, *The Best Friend's™ Approach to Dementia Care*, 2nd ed. (Baltimore, MD: Health Professions Press, 2017).

2. Deborah Barr, MA, Edward G. Shaw, MD, and Gary Chapman, PhD, *Keeping Love Alive as Memories Fade: The 5 Love Languages® and the Alzheimer's Journey*, (Chicago: Northfield Publishing, 2016).

3. Our Rabbi Jesus: His Jewish Life and Teaching, "Hesed: Love in the Long Term," accessed November 2, 2018, http://ourrabbijesus.com/articles/hesed_love_long_term.

4. Carl Rogers, "The attitude and orientation of the counselor in client-centered therapy," *Journal of Consulting Psychology* 13 no. 2, (1949): 82–94.

5. Tom Kitwood, *Dementia Reconsidered: The Person Comes First* (Maidenhead: Open University Press, 1997).

6. See note 5 above, page 40–41.

7. See note 5 above, page 16.

8. World Health Organization, *WHO global strategy on people-centred and integrated health services: Interim report* (Geneva, Switzerland: World Health Organization, 2015).

9. Institute of Medicine Committee on Quality of Health Care in America, *Crossing the Quality Chasm: A New Health System for the 21st Century* (Washington, DC: National Academy Press, 2001).

10. Organisation for Economic Co-Operation and Development, *Addressing Dementia: The OECD Response, OECD Health Policy Studies* (Paris: OECD Publishing, 2015).

11. Sam Fazio, PhD, Douglas Pace, NHA, Katie Maslow, MSW, Sheryl Zimmerman, PhD, and Beth Kallmyer, MSW, "Alzheimer's Association Dementia Care Practice Recommendations," *The Gerontologist*, 58 no. S1 (2018): S1–S9, https://doi:10.1093/geront/gnx182.

12. See note 11 above.

13. Alzheimer's Association, "Dementia Care Practice Recommendations," https://www.alz.org/professionals/professional-providers/dementia_ care_practice_recommendations.

14. Sheila L Molony, PhD, APRN, GNP-BC Ann Kolanowski, PhD, RN, FGSA, FAAN Kimberly Van Haitsma, PhD, and Kate E Rooney, DNP APRN, AGPCNP-BC, "Person-centered assessment and care planning," The Gerontologist 58 no. S1 (2018): S32–S47, https://doi.org/10.1093/geront/gnx173.

Chapter 5: Treatment

1. Dale E. Bredesen, MD, *The End of Alzheimer's: The First Program to Prevent and Reverse Cognitive Decline* (New York: Avery, 2017).

2. Being Patient, "What Does the End of Alzheimer's Mean?" https://www.beingpatient.com/dale-bredesen-end-of-alzheimers/.

3. Ayesha and Dean Sherzai, MD, *The Alzheimer's Solution: A Breakthrough Program to Prevent and Reverse the Symptoms of Cognitive Decline at Every Age* (New York: Harper Collins Publishers, 2017).

4. Jeffrey L. Cummings, Garam Lee, Aaron Ritter, and Kate Zhong, "Alzheimer's disease drug development pipeline: 2018," Alzheimer's & Dementia: Translational Research & Clinical Interventions, 4 (2018): 195–214, https://www.ncbi.nlm.nih.gov/pubmed/29955663.

5. See note 4 above.

6. See note 1 above, page 91.

7. See note 1 above, page 26.

8. See note 1 above, page 6–7.

9. Richard Furman, MD, *Defeating Dementia: What You Can Do to Prevent Alzheimer's and Other Forms of Dementia* (Grand Rapids, MI: Revell, 2018).

10. See note 3 above, pages 14–19.

11. David Gorski, "Functional medicine: The ultimate misnomer in the world of integrative medicine," Science-Based Medicine, posted April 11, 2016.

12. Alzheimer's Disease International, *World Alzheimer's Report 2018— The State of the Art of Dementia Research: New Frontiers*, https://www. alz.co.uk/research/WorldAlzheimerReport2018.pdf.

Chapter 6: Experimental Trials

1. David Watson, Psy.D., personal communication, February 21, 2020.

2. United States Government Accountability Office (GAO), *Report to Congressional Requesters—Drug Industry: Profits, Research, and Development Spending and Merger and Acquisition Deals* (Washington, DC: GAO, November 2017), 18–40.

3. See note 1 above.

4. Ben Readhead, Jean-Vianney Haure-Mirande, Cory C. Funk, Matthew A. Richards, Paul Shannon, Vahram Haroutunian, Mary Sano, Winnie S. Liang, Noam D. Beckmann, Nathan D. Price, Eric M. Reiman, Eric E. Schadt, Michelle E. Ehrlich, Sam Gandy, and Joel T. Dudley, "Multiscale Analysis of Independent Alzheimer's Cohorts Finds Disruption of Molecular, Genetic, and Clinical Networks by Human Herpesvirus," *Neuron*, 99 (2018) https://doi:10.1016/j.neuron.2018.05.023.

5. Robert Tycko, "Molecular Structure of Aggregated Amyloid-β: Insights from Solid-State Nuclear Magnetic Resonance," *Cold Spring Harbor Perspectives in Medicine* 6 no. 8 (2016), https://www.ncbi.nlm.nih.gov/pmc/articles/PMC4968170/.

6. Bill Gates, "Why diagnosing Alzheimer's today is so difficult— and how we can do it better," *GatesNotes: The Blog of Boll Gates*, posted July 17, 2018, https://www.gatesnotes.com/Health/A-better-way-of-diagnosing-Alzheimers.

7. Craig Ritchie, Tom C. Russ, Surjo Banerjee, Bob Barber, Andrew Boaden, Nick C. Fox, Clive Holmes, Jeremy D. Isaacs, Iracema Leroi, Simon Lovestone, Matt Norton, John O'Brien, Jim Pearson, Richard Perry, James Pickett, Adam D. Waldman, Wai Lup Wong, Martin Rossor, and Alistair Burns, "The Edinburgh Consensus: Preparing for the Advent of Disease-modifying Therapies for Alzheimer's Disease," *Alzheimer's Research & Therapy* 9 no. 1 (2017) https://alzres. biomedcentral.com/articles/10.1186/s13195-017-0312-4.

Chapter 7: Care

1. Nancy L. Mace, MA, and Peter V. Rabins, MD, MPH, *The 36-Hour Day: A Family Guide to Caring for People Who Have Alzheimer's Disease, Related Dementias, and Memory Loss, 5th ed.*, (New York: Grand Central Life & Style, 2011)

2. Our Rabbi Jesus: His Jewish Life and Teaching, "Hesed: Love in the Long Term," accessed November 2, 2018, http://ourrabbijesus.com/ articles/hesed_love_long_term.

3. Alzheimer's Association, "2015 Alzheimer's Disease Facts and Figures," *Alzheimer's and Dementia*, 11 no. 3 (2015): 332–384. https://doi. org/10.1016/j.jalz.2015.02.003.

4. National Institutes of Health, National Institute on Aging, "Legal and Financial Planning for People with Alzheimer's," https://www.nia.nih. gov/health/legal-and-financial-planning-people-alzheimers.

5. E Jutkowitz, R.L. Kane, J.E. Gaugler, R.F. MacLehose, B. Dowd, and K.M. Kuntz, "Societal and Family Lifetime Cost of Dementia: Implications for Policy," *Journal of American Geriatric Society*, 65(10) (2017), 2169–75.

6. A.S. Kelley, K. McGarry, R. Gorges, and J.S. Skinner, "The Burden of Health Care Costs for Patients with Dementia in the Last 5 Years of Life," *Annals of Internal Medicine*,163 (2015), 729–36.

7. Steven A. Sass, "How Medicaid helps older Americans," *Issue in Brief* 18-5 (2018), http://hdl.handle.net/2345/bc-ir:107910.

8. Centers for Medicare and Medicaid Services (CMS), "State Operations Manual—Chapter 2: The Certification Process," https://www.cms.gov/Regulations-and-Guidance/Guidance/Manuals/Downloads/som107c02.pdf.

9. See note 8 above, Section 2180c.

10. Centers for Disease Control and Prevention (CDC), "QuickStats: Percentage Distribution of Adult Day Services Centers, by Type of Service—National Study of Long-Term Care Providers, 2016," *Morbidity and Mortality Weekly Report, MMWR*, 67 no. 32 (2016), doi:10.15585/mmwr.mm6732a8.

11. V. Rome, L.D. Harris-Kojetin, and E. Park-Lee, "Variation in Operating Characteristics of Adult Day Services Centers, by Center Ownership: United States, 2014," NCHS Data Brief, No. 224 (2015), 1–8.

12. Genworth, "Genworth Cost of Care Survey 2019: Median Cost Data Tables," https://pro.genworth.com/riiproweb/productinfo/pdf/282102.pdf.

13. United States Department of Health and Human Services, Office of the Assistant Secretary for Planning and Evaluation (ASPE), "Regulatory Review of Adult Day Services Final Report: 2014 Edition, December 1, 2014," https://aspe.hhs.gov/basic-report/regulatory-review-adult-day-services-final-report-2014-edition.

14. Justice in Aging, "Training to Serve People with Dementia: Is Our Health Care System Ready?" https://www.justiceinaging.org/wp-content/uploads/2015/08/Training-to-serve-people-with-dementia-Alz2FINAL.pdf.

15. See note 12 above.

16. L. Harris-Kojetin, M. Sengupta, E. Park-Lee, R. Valverde, C. Caffrey, V. Rome, et al., "Long-term care providers and services users in the United States: Data from the National Study of Long-Term Care

Providers," 2013–2014, National Center for Health Statistics, Vital Health Stat 3 2016;(38):x–xii;1–105.

17. H.M. Arrighi, P.J. Neumann, I.M. Lieberburg, R.J. Townsend, "Lethality of Alzheimer disease and its impact on nursing home placement," *Alzheimer's Disease and Associated Disorders*, 24(1) (2010), 90–95.

18. See note 12 above.

19. Hollis Turnham, Esq., "Federal Nursing Home Reform Act from the Omnibus Budget Reconciliation Act of 1987—OBRA '87 SUMMARY," https://www.ncmust.com/doclib/OBRA87summary.pdf.

20. Centers for Medicare and Medicaid Services (CMS), "Medicare and Medicaid Programs; Reform of Requirements for Long-Term Care Facilities," *Federal Register*, October 4, 2016, https://www.federalregister.gov/documents/2016/10/04/2016-23503/medicare-and-medicaid-programs-reform-of-requirements-for-long-term-care-facilities.

21. See note 12 above.

22. Alzheimer's Association, "2018 Alzheimer's Disease Facts and Figures," https://www.alz.org/media/documents/alzheimers-facts-and-figures-infographic.pdf.

23. Merck, KGaA, *The 2017 Carers Report: Embracing the Critical Role of Caregivers Around the World—White Paper and Action Plan*, October 2017, https://www.embracingcarers.com/content/dam/web/healthcare/corporate/embracing-carers/media/infographics/us/Merck%20KGaA%20Embracing%20Carers_White%20Paper%20Flattened.pdf.

24. World Health Organization (WHO), "Global action plan on the public health response to dementia 2017–2025," http://apps.who.int/iris/bitstream/handle/10665/259615/9789241513487-eng.pdf;jsessionid=D32E69D120DFC4F9607448CDD4F88B7D?sequence=1.

25. Alzheimer's Disease International (ADI), "Principles of a dementia-friendly community," https://www.alz.co.uk/dementia-friendly-communities/principles.

Chapter 8: Hospice

1. National Institutes of Health: National Institute on Aging, "What are Palliative Care and Hospice Care?" https://www.nia.nih.gov/health/what-are-palliative-care-and-hospice-care.

2. American Academy of Hospice and Palliative Medicine and Health Workforce Institute and George Washington University, "A Profile of New Hospice and Palliative Medicine Physicians: Results from the Survey of Hospice and Palliative Medicine Fellows Who Completed Training in 2018," January 2019, http://aahpm.org/uploads/Profile_of_New_HPM_Physicians_2018_June_2019.pdf.

3. Lydia Zuraw, "As Palliative Care Needs Grow, Specialists Are Scarce," NPR, April 5, 2013, https://www.npr.org/sections/health-shots/2013/04/03/176121044/as-palliative-care-need-grows-specialists-are-scarce.

4. World Health Organization (WHO), "Palliative Care," updated February 19, 2018, http://www.who.int/news-room/fact-sheets/detail/palliative-care.

5. Center to Advance Palliative Care (CAPC) and National Palliative Care Research Center, "*America's Care of Serious Illness: A State-by-State Report Card on Access to Palliative Care in Our Nation's Hospitals*," 2019, https://reportcard.capc.org/wp-content/uploads/2015/08/CAPC-Report-Card-2015.pdf.

6. National Consensus Project for Quality Palliative Care and National Coalition for Hospice and Palliative Care, *Clinical Practice Guidelines for Quality Palliative Care* (4th ed.), 2018, https://www.nationalcoalitionhpc.org/wp-content/uploads/2018/10/NCHPC-NCPGuidelines_4thED_web_FINAL.pdf.

7. National Hospice and Palliative Care Organization, "Hospice Care," https://www.nhpco.org/about/hospice-care-overview.

8. National Hospice and Palliative Care Organization, *Facts and Figures: 2018 Edition*, https://www.nhpco.org/wp-content/uploads/2019/07/2018_NHPCO_Facts_Figures.pdf.

9. Centers for Medicare and Medicaid Services, *Medicare Hospice Benefits*, https://www.medicare.gov/Pubs/pdf/02154-Medicare-Hospice-Benefits.PDF.

10. "Hospice Compare," Medicare, https://www.medicare.gov/hospicecompare.

Chapter 9: Death

1. World Health Organization (WHO), "The Top Ten Causes of Death," May 24, 2018, http://www.who.int/en/news-room/fact-sheets/detail/the-top-10-causes-of-death.

2. World Life Expectancy, "World Health Rankings," https://www.worldlifeexpectancy.com/cause-of-death/alzheimers-dementia/by-country.

3. Office for National Statistics, "Deaths Registered in England and Wales (series DR): 2017," https://www.ons.gov.uk/peoplepopulationandcommunity/birthsdeathsandmarriages/deaths/bulletins/deathsregisteredinenglandandwalesseriesdr/2017.

4. Heron M. "Deaths: Leading causes for 2016," National Vital Statistics Reports, vol 67 no 6. Hyattsville, MD: National Center for Health Statistics. 2018, https://www.cdc.gov/nchs/data/nvsr/nvsr67/nvsr67_06.pdf.

5. Centers for Disease Control and Prevention (CDC), "Disease of the Week: Alzheimer's Disease," https://www.cdc.gov/dotw/alzheimers/.

6. WebMD, "What to Expect When Your Loved One is Dying," https://www.webmd.com/palliative-care/journeys-end-active-dying#1.

7. National Institute on Aging, "What to Do After Someone Dies," https://www.nia.nih.gov/health/what-do-after-someone-dies.
8. National Institute on Aging, "Alzheimer's Disease Research Centers," https://www.nia.nih.gov/health/alzheimers-disease-research-centers.
9. National Institute on Aging, "Brain Donation Resources for ADRCs," https://www.nia.nih.gov/health/brain-donation-resources-adrcs.
10. National Institutes of Health (NIH), "NeuroBioBank," https://neurobiobank.nih.gov/about/#network.

Chapter 10: Grief

1. Elisabeth Kübler-Ross, MD and David Kessler, *On Grief and Grieving: Finding the Meaning of Grief Through the Five Stages of Loss* (New York: Scribner, 2005).
2. The Center for Complicated Grief, "Overview," https://complicatedgrief.columbia.edu/professionals/complicated-grief-professionals/overview.
3. Mayo Clinic, "Complicated Grief," https://www.mayoclinic.org/diseases-conditions/complicated-grief/symptoms-causes/syc-20360374.
4. See note 1 above.

ACKNOWLEDGMENTS

There are people who really were care angels in Mom's life during her illness. These are the people I want to thank from the bottom of my heart:

Thank you, Malisa Huxable, for caring for and loving Mom, and looking after me, too, when we needed an angel like you the most.

Thank you, Meredith LaPira, President of Home Care Assistance (HCA) of South Florida, for placing Malisa with Mom, for caring for Mom and visiting her when she was in the hospital, and for leading HCA with your heart. The industry needs to clone you.

Thank you, Dr. Jose Conde of the Medical Associates of Delray practice, for caring for and about Mom throughout her illness and for giving sound and compassionate advice.

Thank you, to the Jade hospice team with Trustbridge in Florida. Everyone on that team was so caring, loving, and gentle with Mom.

Thank you, Sue Gervase and Sandra Holden, for your help in caring for Mom and for the love you showed her.

I also want to thank my husband, Jim, who picked up his life without a second thought so that he and I could live with Mom and care for her. He continues to be the person I lean on when my knees still buckle.

My brother, David, his wife, Sheri, and their two girls, Randi and Jamie, know how much Mom loved them, and how much I love them. I know it is not necessary to say "thank you" to them, and they would not want me to, but I do want to acknowledge a few things. David, you were Mom's rock throughout much of her life, and you always brought her joy and made her laugh. Sheri, you were a daughter to Mom, and are still a sister to me. I am looking forward to the years to come in our rocking chairs on the front porch. Randi and Jamie, you gave Mom more joy than anyone could for all the years of your life.

My sister, Erin, her husband, Chet, and son, Anthony, were challenged with not living in the same state as Mom during this difficult time. But they were always in Mom's heart, as she was in theirs. Mom's joy and contentment showed on her face when she was with you. She loved you all so much.

Thank you, Lisa and Rick Park, for your steadfast and lifelong friendship. And, Lisa, thank you for being there for me so many days when I needed you after Mom passed, and for all your help reviewing this book.

I also had a dear friend, Toby Vitek, who lost her own life to cancer almost a year after Mom passed away and whose mother had Alzheimer's too. Toby spent many hours on the phone with me helping me understand what I might expect. Toby is missed and loved.

Finally, I want to thank the team at PYP Press, who are a great group of people and really care about helping you bring your passion alive through the words on the page. I could not have finished this book without Jenn, Niki, Karen, and the rest of the PYP team.

PLEASE HELP TO ADVANCE COMMUNICATION AND EDUCATION REGARDING ALZHEIMER'S

You can order more copies of this book at your favorite book retailer or through our website at www.AlzheimersMatters.com. Please give one to your family and friends who are impacted by this terrible disease. And please don't forget to provide a review for the book.

Also visit www.AlzheimersMatters.com to learn more about the company, Alzheimer's Matters™, and to get on our mailing list. On the website, you will find resources on various topics related to the disease. Through the website, we also conduct many surveys to collect information from family caregivers in order to learn more about the disease and caring for someone with the disease.

Dr. Terri Baumgardner also speaks to various audiences about Alzheimer's disease—particularly topics related to caregiving. You can book her for conferences, community groups and forums, business education forums, etc., through the company website or by emailing the company at info@alzheimersmatters.com.

To stay up to date on our current work and events, please follow Alzheimer's Matters™ on Twitter (@AlzMatters), Facebook at https://www.facebook.com/AlzheimersMatters/ and Instagram at https://www.instagram.com/alzheimersmatters/.

ABOUT THE AUTHOR

Dr. Terri Baumgardner has spent her 28-year career working with executives around the world to be stronger leaders, build more effective organizations, and handle challenges with aplomb, integrity, and grace. With a Ph.D. in Industrial/ Organizational psychology, her career has included overseeing geographic regions of an international leadership and talent consulting firm, leading the 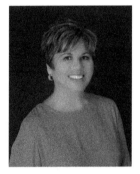 strategic talent management and organizational effectiveness function for a Fortune 50 organization, and founding and leading two companies.

As an expert in leadership and talent in organizations, she has published a number of book chapters and journal articles and presented for corporate audiences and at professional conferences. Dr. Baumgardner has also worked as an adjunct professor, teaching graduate students in MBA and Organizational Leadership master's programs in business and psychology departments of several universities. She has taught courses in Leadership, Talent Management, Human Resources Management, Organizational Behavior, Strategy and Execution, and Leadership Communication. With an additional master's degree in communication and journalism, she also works with leaders on improving communications.

Over two years ago, after caring for her mother—who had Alzheimer's disease for several years—and having a grandmother and two uncles who also died with the disease, she founded her second company, Alzheimer's Matters™. Its mission is to advance communication, education, and quality of care related to Alzheimer's disease and other dementias. This book represents one of the efforts to improve understanding regarding Alzheimer's and dementia.

Dr. Baumgardner has spent a career helping leaders to be exceptional. She is now expanding her focus and determination to help people suffering from Alzheimer's and other dementias, and those who love and care for them. Visit her companies' websites to find out more, at www.sarbergardner.com and www.alzheimersmatters.com.

CPSIA information can be obtained
at www.ICGtesting.com
Printed in the USA
LVHW071638121021
700248LV00013B/234/J